Health & environmental impact assessment

An integrated approach

Health & environmental impact assessment

An integrated approach

British Medical Association

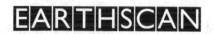

Earthscan Publications Ltd, London

First published in the UK in 1998 by
Earthscan Publications Ltd

Reprinted 1999

Copyright © British Medical Association, 1998

A catalogue record for this book is available from the British Library

ISBN: 1 85383 541 2 (paperback)
ISBN: 1 85383 540 4 (hardback)

Typesetting by Hilary Glanville

Page design by Paul Sands, S&W Design

Text photographs: pages 65 (bottom), 113 © BMA News Review; pages 18, 23, 46, 78, 146, 147, 151 © Environment Agency; pages 61, 63, 65 (top), 66, 67, 69, 76, 107, 110, 114, 117, 119, 120, 122, 124 © Alexis Maryon; pages 4, 11 © Rural Development Commission.

Printed and bound by Biddles Ltd, Guildford and King's Lynn

Cover design by Hilary Glanville and Yvonne Booth
Cover photograph © David Nunuk/Science Photo Library

For a full list of Earthscan publications, please contact
Earthscan Publications Ltd
120 Pentonville Road
London N1 9JN
Tel: 0171 278 0433
Fax: 0171 278 1142
email: earthinfo@earthscan.co.uk
http://www.earthscan.co.uk

For details of BMA Science publications, please contact:
BMJ BOOKSHOP
BMA House
Tavistock Square
London WC1H 9JR
Tel: 0171 383 6244/6638
Fax: 0171 383 6662
http://www.bma.org.uk

Earthscan is an editorially independent subsidiary of Kogan Page Limited and publishes in association with WWF-UK and the International Institute for Environment and Development.

Contents

List of figures

List of tables

Working Party

A working party with the following membership was set up to advise the Board of Science and Education.

Professor S T Holgate (Chairman)	MRC Clinical Professor of Immunopharmacology, University of Southampton
Professor H R Anderson	Professor of Epidemiology and Public Health, St George's Hospital Medical School
Professor J G Ayres	Professor of Respiratory Medicine, Birmingham Heartlands Hospital and University of Warwick
Dr N Olsen	Member of the BMA Board of Science and Education, Independent Public Health Physician, Newton Ferrers, Devon
Dr D Osborn	Head of Pollution and Ecotoxicology Section, Natural Environment Research Council Institute of Terrestrial Ecology
Mr S D Price	Group Manager Emissions and Pollution, Highways Agency, Executive Agency of the Department of Transport

Acknowledgements

The Association is indebted to the Working Party members for so generously giving of their time and expertise and is particularly grateful for the specialist help provided by the BMA Committees and many outside experts and organisations, and would particularly like to thank:

Professor D J Ball, Director, School of Health, Biological and Environmental Sciences, Middlesex University; Dr J Beach, Institute of Occupational Health, University of Birmingham; Professor D Coggon, MRC Environmental Epidemiology Unit, University of Southampton; Dr P T C Harrison, MRC Institute for Environment and Health, University of Leicester; Mr G Jukes, Chartered Institute of Environmental Health.

Approval for publication as a BMA policy report was recommended by BMA Council on 1 October 1997.

CHAPTER 1

Introduction

The British Medical Association

The British Medical Association (BMA) is a professional organisation representing all doctors in the UK. It was established in 1832 *to promote the medical and allied sciences, and to maintain the honour and interests of the medical profession.* The BMA Board of Science and Education supports this aim by providing an interface between the profession, the government, and the public. By undertaking research studies on behalf of the BMA, and through the publication of policy reports, the Board of Science and Education has led the debate on key public health and professional issues.

One major objective of the Board of Science and Education is to contribute to the development of better public health policies that affect the community, the state, and the medical profession. In order to do this, the Board appoints working parties and steering groups, combining medical and other specialist expertise to undertake investigations to examine the impact of various policies and activities on public health. The Board has published a number of reports over recent years, reflecting current concerns, such as pesticide toxicity, transport policy, complementary medicine, bloodborne infections, and the environmental and occupational risks of health care[1,2,3,4,5] and has developed BMA policy in a range of medico-sociological topic areas.

The Board is also responsible for developing educational initiatives. Some of the reports and video presentations published through the Board have been used in medical education programmes, in secondary schools and in higher education. The Board not only develops such educational materials, but also has an interest in educational policy, and has examined the education of doctors in clinical safety, multicultural health care, and other issues.

BMA policy on the environment

The BMA has produced a number of policy documents which focus on aspects of environmental health and pollution and which recommend policies for national action by government, other organisations and individuals, with specific recommendations affecting the medical and allied professions. In 1987 the BMA published *Living with Risk*,[6] a comprehensive guide which explored the risks associated with the environment as part of a wide ranging investigation into how individuals perceive, manage and prevent risk. *Pesticides, Chemicals and Health*[7] examined the current need for the use of pesticides, reviewed the literature concerning acute and chronic effects on human health, methods of control and surveillance, and alternatives to chemical pesticides. *Hazardous Waste and Human Health*[8] provided an overview of the existing evidence relating to the adverse health effects due to exposure to hazardous waste. This evidence was presented in relation to the characteristics of hazardous waste, its origins, disposal methods and regulations governing the management of waste.

The BMA's Board of Science and Education has considered air pollution caused by the internal combustion engine and recommendations for actions to reduce pollution were published in the report *Cycling: toward health and safety*.[9] The report recommended the active promotion of cycling as an environmentally friendly means of transport, and suggested ways in which cycling could be made safer and more accessible. In a further report, *Road Transport and Health*[10] published in 1997, the BMA highlighted the many ways in which transport policy can affect health, considering not only the more obvious effects such as accidents and pollution but also other consequences of transport policy such as the decline in public transport services, particularly in rural areas, the lowering of the quality of life in inner-city residents and the associated lack of physical activity leading to unhealthy lifestyles. In 1994 the Board of Science and Education reviewed the issues surrounding water disconnections and the effects on individual and public health.[11] Also in 1994 the BMA addressed concerns over the adverse effects of medical technology through publication of a report on *Environmental and Occupational Risks of Health Care*.[12] The report considered risks to health and the environment from chemicals, radiation, infectious agents and disposal of clinical waste as well as numerous other processes carried out as part of health care. Further guidance on clinical waste, storage and disposal has been given by the Association through its *Code of practice for the safe use and disposal of sharps*[13] and the *Code of practice for sterilisation of instruments and control of cross infection.*[14]

Doctors, human health and the environment

The medical profession has an important role to play in exploring risks to human health so that hazards can be controlled, diminished or eliminated. A key practical recommendation that arose from the BMA's work regarding the environment called for doctors to "play an active part in managing the environment in the interests of public health".[15]

In recent years, with growing public interest in environmental issues, increasing concern has been shown over the environmental consequences of unrestrained environmental development. This has resulted in the introduction of new national and international legislation intended to safeguard the environment and promote sustainability. Environmental impact assessment is one such example which has been legislated for in many countries, to ensure that environmental effects are taken fully into account when planning new development. New development can have major implications for human health, both on a national, local and individual basis. The health and quality of life of people depend substantially on the physical, social, economic and commercial environment in which they live. This environment is increasingly compromised by human activity and there are few areas of the world left which are completely unaffected by the direct or indirect effect of humans. Much recent development has been enormously beneficial to human life and for many the quality of their built environment, their food and water supply and their employment and leisure activities bring them a quality and duration of life unmatched in history. Unfortunately, the increase in the population and the consumption of natural resources to achieve this are now widely recognised as unsustainable. As more and more parts of the world become industrialised and energy and material consumption increase, the problems will be aggravated. In an environment where scant regard is paid to the precautionary principle (see section 4.4.5) or to the desirability of some proposed development, and where its potential profitability is the dominant or sole

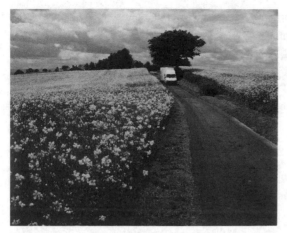

Rape fields may exacerbate pollen allergy

consideration, market forces can have serious adverse effects on environmental and public health.

In addition to the health impact assessment of development projects, there is a need to assess the health impacts, both positive and negative, of policies. One example is agricultural policy which can have a health impact through food standards, access to food, and nutritional status of the population, as well as other implications such as the planting of rape seed which may have an adverse health impact for those who are allergic to pollen.

Government departments, other organisations or agencies often send consultation documents to the BMA for consideration and comment on the medical/health aspects of the document. This consultation exercise could be considered to be a preliminary health impact assessment. Issues may arise from this preliminary review which could indicate that a detailed health impact assessment needs to be carried out. A full health impact assessment may be a very detailed piece of work, and at present the methodology is at an early developmental stage. The BMA believes that a framework for regulation is required to enable the assessment of development projects and public policies to be undertaken within a wider strategic set of objectives which contribute to the overall goal of sustainability, and maintenance of health.

Human health is determined by a number of factors including genetic predisposition, lifestyle, nutrition, socio-economic status, access to adequate health care, and the environment. The multidimensional nature of human health was emphasised in 1995 by the BMA report *Inequalities in Health*[16] which noted that the quality of the environment affects all sectors of society, especially those in deprived groups. The continuing availability of environmental resources — air, water, food and shelter — as well as appropriate climatic and socio-economic conditions, is a prerequisite for health and survival. Environmental conditions are not always optimal however, and populations may be exposed to a variety of environmental factors that may adversely affect their health and wellbeing. These environmental hazards may result from natural causes and/or human activities. Healthy environments and healthy populations are therefore interdependent.

Despite this clear interdependence, the protection of human health and the environment have traditionally been addressed separately, through the provision of health care services and public health legislation on the one hand, and through environmental protection measures on the other. At various times, especially since the 1970s, references have been made to the importance of relationships between the environmental and health sectors, but in practice little progress has been made towards their integrated assessment and regulation. In 1996, however, the professional body which represents Environmental Health Officers, the Chartered Institute of Environmental Health, established an Environmental Health Commission in collaboration with the Royal Environmental Health Institute of Scotland, and the city councils of Edinburgh and Oxford. The conclusions of that Commission were published in July 1997.[17] The Commission concluded that human beings can only be healthy in a healthy environment, and provided a set of detailed recommendations for institutional and policy reforms, including the need for local authorities to develop techniques for integrated environmental health impact assessment. These recommendations can be expected to contribute to improving both environmental and public health.

At the BMA Annual Representative Meeting in 1994, there was a debate on impact assessment in the UK. A resolution was passed calling upon the BMA Board of Science and Education to *review the methods for health impact assessment of environmental projects, and then press the government to undertake them for all major projects affecting the environment.* As a result of this debate, a preliminary report was prepared for the Board of Science and Education by Dr D Osborn of the Natural Environment Research Council (NERC) which formed the basis for discussion at an informal round table meeting held in June 1995. Following the meeting, a formal BMA working party was established to examine the degree of emphasis given to the dynamic relationship between human and environmental health in the light of existing public health legislation, health care provision and formal environmental assessment procedures. The outcome of this study and recommendations formed the basis for this report.

Aims, scope and structure of the report

This present report further develops the BMA's policies on health and the environment. One of its aims is to challenge the way people think about impact assessment both at a national/strategic and local/project level and to set out what is known, and what remains to be learnt about the process of environmental impact assessment (EIA), and to show how this might be enhanced.

The report considers actions that could potentially affect the environment and human health. Such actions may be individual development proposals submitted for planning consent, or proposals for plans, policies or programmes. For terminological convenience the text will refer primarily to 'projects', although policies, programmes and plans are included, except where otherwise stated. The environmental impacts of these are addressed through project-level environmental impact assessment (EIA) and strategic environmental assessment (SEA) respectively. The assessment of health impacts may be addressed through health impact assessment (HIA) with respect to either project-level EIA or strategic-level SEA. These various forms of assessment are described in detail in Chapter 3.

Provisions for the assessment of health impacts within EIA vary between countries. Mandatory provision for SEA is in place in a relatively small number of countries, but there is ongoing consultation on a European SEA Directive.[18] This report refers primarily to existing EU and UK legislation, but also summarises experience from developing countries. Drawing on this experience, together with some UK examples and case studies taken from earlier BMA policy documents, the report considers the need for integrated health and environmental impact assessment and suggests ways in which HIA could be incorporated more explicitly into the existing UK EIA procedures. This is particularly important since the European Commission has clarified that Article 129 of the Treaty on the European Union "requires the Commission to check that proposals for policies, and implementation measures and instruments, do not have an adverse impact on health, or create conditions which undermine the promotion of health".[19] Despite this commitment to health impact assessment, there is, at present, no systematic means by which this requirement can be implemented. The report draws attention to the need for future developments in this field to encompass prospective assessment of the health impact of policies, programmes and plans.

The contribution to be made by epidemiologists, toxicologists and others is discussed, and reference is made to the role of health outcome measurement by health economists. In particular, it is noted that although many parallels exist between health impact assessment and methods of evaluation used in health economics, health economists have, to date, focused almost exclusively on health care interventions rather than non-health sector policies that affect health. It can be argued that health economists will need to extend their scope beyond the remedial health sector in order to contribute not only to policies for remedial health care, but more broadly to policies for the maintenance and promotion of health.

Pure human resource development programmes, such as teacher training and the evaluation of health sector projects, such as a new hospital, are specialist subjects and will not be examined specifically. Furthermore, projects which have health improvements as their main objective, such as improved safety features in cars, are outside the scope of this report.

The report is aimed at both the general and professional reader. It will be particularly valuable to those responsible for environmental and health impact assessment who do not need to be experts (for example in occupational and public health, water supply engineering or traffic management), but who do need to ensure that appropriate expertise is consulted as necessary. It provides useful background information for a wide range of professionals, including medical practitioners, environmental health officers, town planners, and local councillors in making decisions about development projects. It should also be of interest to the general reader who is concerned about decisions which may have an impact on their health and/or the amenity of their environment, or those who simply wish to know more about this subject.

Chapter 1 sets out the aims and objectives of the report, within the context of past BMA policy relating to the role of doctors in protecting human and environmental health.

Chapter 2 examines ways of managing the environment to safeguard human health. The current UK institutional framework for protecting the environment and health is explored within the broader concept of sustainable development. The chapter concludes with a look at how current planning of new developments fits into this institutional framework.

Chapter 3 outlines the development and current provision of environmental impact assessment in the UK, including its origins in European legislation. The potential for strategic impact assessment of policies, programmes and plans is also considered. Health impact assessment is introduced as a methodology which aims to identify, predict and evaluate the likely changes in health risk of a development action on a defined population. Evidence from a previously unpublished pilot study is presented to show that UK impact assessments frequently gave insufficient consideration to possible health impacts.

Chapter 4 proposes a methodology for the integration of health within the various stages of the environmental impact assessment process. Three key stages are discussed: the identification of health hazards; the interpretation of health hazards as health risks; and the management of health risks. Examples and case studies relating to the application of health impact assessment for a range of projects and policies in the UK are presented.

Chapter 5 looks at the wider social and economic issues including scope for interdisciplinary collaboration. The methodological guiding principles needed to achieve effective health impact assessment are outlined, with a warning about the consequences of ignoring health impact.

Chapter 6 summarises the findings and conclusions of the report and makes a number of recommendations to take these forward in the form of policies for the next millennium. The recommendations address areas such as national policies, the corporate sector, the future design and conduct of impact assessments, decision-making, research, education and training.

2

Management of the environment to safeguard human health: the background

Defining the environment

Einstein once remarked: "the environment is everything which isn't me".[1] In its broadest sense, the word 'environment' embraces all the conditions or influences under which any individual or thing exists, lives or develops. Peace and social stability is clearly an underlying condition, the importance of which was brought into sharp focus by the BMA report on the medical and health impacts of nuclear war.[2] The environment can be distinguished under several headings. Gilpin[3] has divided these into three sets:

- the combination of physical conditions that affect and influence the growth and development of an individual or community;
- the social, cultural and economic conditions that affect the nature of an individual or community;
- the surrounding of an inanimate object of intrinsic social value.

The environment of human beings can also be categorised into:

- the abiotic factors such as the land, the water, the atmosphere, climate, sounds, odours and tastes;
- the biotic factors including other human beings, as well as the fauna, flora, ecology, bacteria, and viruses; and
- all of those social factors which together constitute the quality of our lives.

The UK Strategy on Sustainable Development defines the word 'environment' as "external conditions or surroundings in which people, plants and animals live, which tend to influence their development and behaviour. ... environment is taken to relate to natural media - air, water, soil, land and natural resources - landscape and the countryside, and man-made developments such as buildings and roads".[4] Gilpin's (1995) account of the constituents of the "environment" are reflected in most national legislative regimes, and this is represented in Table 1.[5]

Table 1: Ingredients of the word 'environment' as reflected in most national legislation	
All aspects of the surroundings of human beings, whether affecting human beings as individuals or in social groupings	✓
Natural resources including air, land and water	✓
Ecosystems and biological diversity	✓
Social, economic, and cultural circumstances	✓
Infrastructure and associated equipment	✓
Any solid, liquid, gas, odour, heat, noise, vibration, or radiation resulting directly or indirectly from the activities of human beings	✓
Identified natural assets such as natural beauty, outlooks, and scenic routes	✓
Identified historical and heritage assets	✓
Identified cultural and religious assets	✓
Aesthetic assets	✓
Public health characteristics	✓
Identifiable environmental planning, environmental protection, environmental management, pollution control, nature conservation, and other mitigation measures	✓

Sustainability

The concept of sustainability was famously and succinctly defined by the World Commission on Environment and Development[6] as development which "meets the needs of the present without compromising the ability of future generations to meet their own needs". Human health and well-being have had a central position in the interpretation of this concept of sustainability. The UN Conference on Environment and Development[7] declared that "human beings are at the centre of concern for sustainable development. They are entitled to a healthy and productive life in harmony with nature". Any policy, programme or project which compromises human health and well-being cannot, by this definition, be counted as sustainable.

The sustainability of policies, programmes and projects can only be assured if the full range of potential impacts is appraised in a timely fashion and if actions proceed from that appraisal. The potential impacts are numerous and cut across many specialist concerns.[8] The British government published its strategy for sustainable development in January 1994. However, the UN Environment and Development Committee for the UK has pointed out that the 1994 strategy document failed to address major issues concerning the relationship between environment and health.[9] A distinctive feature of the strategy set out

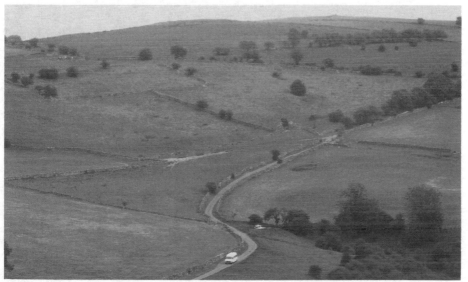

Human beings are entitled to a healthy and productive life in harmony with nature

in Agenda 21 (see Appendix 5) has been a recognition that local government provides the most appropriate forum in which many issues of environmental health and sustainability can best be addressed.[10] The British Government has convened a Panel on Sustainable Development which has criticised the government for not adopting a more pro-active policy in relation to its procurement activities. In other words, the Panel had concluded that when the Government uses public resources to purchase goods and services, it could do more to ensure that those goods and services are produced in a more sustainable fashion. The Panel pointed out that while the government had made a commitment "to make sustainable development the touchstone of its policies", this had not been fully translated into practice.[11,12]

The Panel recommended that the Government should bring the environmental dimension into all its procurement policies to promote sustainable development, and recommended that an evaluation of the environmental policies and practices of all companies bidding for public contracts should become an essential element in all procurement decisions. The BMA has drawn attention to the fact that the health aspects of environmental considerations will be an important ingredient if progress is to be made with making development more sustainable, and has also recommended that public purchasing authorities should try to ensure that purchasing decisions are environmentally sound.[13]

Human health and the environment

Sustainability is obviously essential, but it is not necessarily sufficient. In practice our individual aspirations and public policies should, and often do, aspire to ensuring more than just our survival, but rather that we thrive healthily.

Many impacts on human health are mediated through, or influenced by, the biophysical environment. The nature of potential environmental threats to health varies between countries and is often linked to economic circumstances. There are many health problems which are directly associated with systemic poverty. Lack of water supply infrastructure and poor sanitation, for example, may be associated with high levels of water-borne disease. Over-population in areas where subsistence agriculture is relied on for food supplies may result in widespread malnutrition. The relationship between economic growth and public health is not, however, straightforward. Potential new threats derive from the very technologies which have driven economic growth and industrialisation, and which have enabled us to exploit and control our environment so effectively. The use of energy intensive technologies, combined with high levels of consumption of natural resources results both in the overloading of the environment's capacity to absorb waste and pollution and over-exploitation of natural resources. This progressive depletion of resources and reduction in ability of the environment to contain pollution and waste bring us closer to the carrying capacity of our supporting environment, a situation which A J McMichael[14] refers to as "planetary overload".

It is important to recognise that many environmental threats to human health are trans-boundary and cannot be regulated effectively on a local, regional or even national basis. The effects of the Chernobyl incident, for example, were felt in many countries. We need to be able to measure the overall impacts of development on our surroundings and on ourselves. Human health should be examined within an ecological framework if we are to respond to potential new threats of a global nature, such as pollution-induced climate change.[15] Such threats are more pervasive, complex and harder to understand, avoid and manage than the more localised problems. Historically we have had more experience with problems such as localised pollution incidents, and global environmental problems are altogether more challenging, both technically and politically. In addition, the scale of economic development is now such that localised impacts are beginning to agglomerate. Collectively they may generate cumulative impacts which exceed the sum of their component parts due to synergistic effects.

'Health' in its widest sense incorporates many aspects of human welfare and means much more than simply the absence of disease. The UK Government defines environmental health as "those aspects of human health, including quality of life, that are determined by physical, biological, social and psychosocial factors in the environment. It also refers to the theory and practice of assessing, correcting, controlling and preventing those factors in the environment that can potentially affect adversely the health of present and future generations".[16] This definition emphasises the multi-dimensional nature of health and also the concept of ensuring equity between generations (the guiding principle for sustainable development). The promotion of good health therefore requires not only public policies which support health, but also the creation of supportive environments in which "living and working conditions are safe, stimulating, satisfying and enjoyable".[17]

The complex nature of many modern environmental hazards demands cross-sectoral approaches to safeguarding health, but such approaches are often difficult to organise. There is now a bewildering number of organisations with an interest in health and it is not easy to decide exactly where responsibilities for environmental health do, and should, lie. Ideally, "every public and private body should assess its activities and carry them out in such a way as to protect people's health from harmful effects related to the physical, chemical, biological, microbiological and social environments",[18] but how can accountability for human health consequences of actions be achieved?

Responsibilities for managing the environment to safeguard human health have derived from legislation on public health, occupational and environmental health, the regulation of industrial activity and the planning of new development. (Appendix I outlines key developments in these areas.) Government action to tackle environmental health issues has been both direct and indirect, and voluntary self-regulation of industry has also played a part. In addition to the complexities of managing environmental health issues within countries, there have also been a number of international initiatives to tackle global environmental problems.

UK institutional framework for the protection of the environment and health

The following have important roles and responsibilities in relation to the environmental health consequences of decisions:

- The Government and its Departments
- The Health and Safety Commission (HSC) and Executive (HSE)
- The Environment Agencies (England and Wales, Scotland and Northern Ireland)
- The Royal Commission on Environmental Pollution
- Health Authorities and Directors of Public Health
- Occupational Health Services
- Local authorities
- Non-government organisations and the private sector

The Government and its Departments

There is no single government department responsible for every aspect of environmental health.[19] However, the Secretary of State for the Environment, Transport and the Regions has a general responsibility for environmental protection and coordinates central government activity to ensure that no one part of the environment is controlled at the expense of any other and that an overall view is taken of priorities. There are Cabinet Committees on the Environment and on Health, but there is no Committee with an explicit remit for the consideration of environmental health *per se*. Although issues relevant to environmental health may be raised and discussed in either or both committees, responsibilities for environmental health are less clearly defined than they might be.

In all Government Departments there is a 'Green Minister' with responsibilities to ensure that environmental impacts of their Department's policies and programmes are considered.[20] The 'Green Ministers' meet regularly under the chairmanship of the Environment Minister with the collective aim "to ensure that environmental issues are considered in the development of all government policies to deliver an improved and lasting quality of life". A new Sustainable Development Unit in the Department of the Environment, Transport and the Regions has been introduced to support all Departments in assessing the potential environmental impact of new policy proposals.[21] In spite of this there is no clear framework for addressing complex environmental health issues, particularly those of a cumulative or trans-boundary nature. Central government prepares the statutory framework for environmental protection and issues advice to public pollution control authorities, usually by means of circulars, but also through codes of practice.

In 1992, the Government published the *Health of the Nation* White Paper[22] and set targets for improvements in the nation's health. It recognised that health can be affected by the activities of many public bodies, not only those of the health services, and acknowledged the importance of impact assessment. Recent targets have been outlined in its successor, *Our Healthier Nation*,[23] which has pledged that "...the Government will apply health impact assessments to its relevant key policies, so that when they are being developed and implemented, the consequences of those policies for our health are considered." An interdepartmental working group exists to monitor the work of different government departments in preventing ill-health.

An important step in linking environment and health was taken by the Government in the form of the joint consultation by the Departments of Health and Environment which proposed the addition of 'environment' as a key area within the *Health of the Nation* strategy.[24] The British Medical Association (BMA) welcomed this initiative, but believed that it gave insufficient emphasis to creating environments conducive to promoting improvements in the public health.

Although it is often difficult to measure the influence of poor environment on health, many environmental factors are known, or there are strong reasons to suspect them to be significant causes of, or contributors to, ill-health and reduced quality of life. The failure to assess the health impacts in order to predict and mitigate potential threats to human health is not comprehensively tackled in the *Health of the Nation* strategy,[25,26] or *Our Healthier Nation*.[27] The latter commits the Government to using health impact assessment for relevant key policies, but there are no criteria for deciding relevance, or a strategy of implementation. These matters should be addressed in the final White Paper.

The first Minister of State for Public Health was appointed in 1997. The Minister is responsible for health promotion and public health issues, both generally and within the NHS. These responsibilites include the implementation of the *Health of the Nation* strategy, and its successor, *Our Healthier Nation*, which, at the time of writing, is out for consultation[28] and, importantly includes "the environment and health".[29] This is a key role which places greater priority on human health throughout government, and provides an opportunity to make health impact assessment a routine part of the evaluation of government policies and programmes and existing planning regulations. Further, prospective health impact assessment and auditing of health effects, if carried out after implementation, will provide valuable information on which policy makers and planners can base future decisions.[30]

The Health and Safety Commission and Executive

The Health and Safety Commission (HSC) and Health and Safety Executive (HSE) are "statutory bodies whose aims are to protect the health, safety and welfare of employees and to safeguard others, principally the public, who may be exposed to risks from industrial activity".[31] The HSC is responsible for the administration of the Health and Safety at Work etc Act 1974 and therefore has a key part to play in occupational health concerns. In July 1995, Ministerial responsibility for the HSC and HSE was transferred from the Department of Employment to the Department of the Environment, which later became the Department of the Environment, Transport and the Regions. The HSC is responsible to the Secretary of State for the Environment, Transport and the Regions and other Secretaries of State. The HSE is a distinct statutory body which advises and assists the HSC and has day to day responsibility for enforcing health and safety legislation. Various advisory committees are in place for consultation, especially the Occupational Health Advisory Committee which advises the HSC on:

- encouraging systems for managing health at work;
- developing occupational health services and competencies;
- improving data on occupational disease; and
- promoting health in the workplace.

The Environment Agency

In England and Wales, the Environment Agency (EA) (a non-departmental public body) took over the functions of Her Majesty's Inspectorate of Pollution (HMIP), the National Rivers Authority (NRA) and the local waste regulation authorities, including significant responsibilities for water management as well as pollution control, in 1996. The equivalent agencies in Scotland and Northern Ireland are the Scottish Environment Protection Agency and the Environment and Heritage Service, respectively. The EA represents an important step forward in environmental regulation in the UK, bringing together for the first time the activities of many inter-related agencies to form one of the largest and most powerful environmental regulators in the world. The importance of integration is clearly stated in the EA aims, which are to:

- achieve major and continuous improvements in the quality of air, land and water;
- encourage the conservation of natural resources, animals and plants;
- make the most of pollution control and river-basin management;
- provide effective defence and warning systems to protect people and property against flooding from rivers and the sea;

- reduce the amount of waste by encouraging people to re-use and recycle their waste;
- improve standards of waste disposal;
- manage water resources to achieve the proper balance between the country's needs and the environment;
- work with other organisations to reclaim contaminated land;
- improve and develop salmon and freshwater fisheries;
- conserve and improve river navigation;
- tell people about environmental issues by educating and informing;
- set priorities and work out solutions that society can afford.

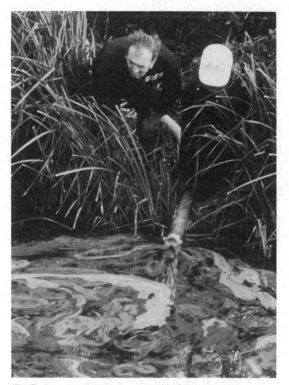

The Environment Agency is responsible for water management and pollution control

The Environment Agency is required and guided by Government to carry out its duties in order to help achieve the objective of sustainable development, at the heart of which is the integration of human needs and the environment. Initially the BMA had criticised the Agency for having an ambiguous view of its role in relation to human and environmental health. Nearly all the functions of the Environment Agency with regard to the protection of the environment ultimately have an impact upon health, and it is this impact that determines the setting of standards and actions required with regard to the environment. The Environment Agency's 1998 strategy document,[32] identifies prevention of harm to human health as part of its principal regulatory function in relation to controlled waste. In addition the Agency will "report regularly on different aspects of the state of the environment ... such as the relationships between the health of the environment and the health of man".

The Agency will undertake a research and development (R&D) programme to support its activities, and will interface with other external R&D programmes. It will provide tools, methodologies, and guidance on environmental monitoring and assessment techniques, which should include contributing to the development of integrated environmental and health impact assessment methodology. The Agency also has a key role to play in monitoring, assessing and advising Government in relation to environmental impacts of pollution and plans to carry out environmental assessments of new and existing chemicals. Such work should provide important data for health and environmental impact assessments.

The Environment Agency also has responsibility for the upkeep and operation of the Chemical Release Inventory (CRI). This is a computerised database set up to record all industrial discharges to the environment that are covered by the provisions of the system of Integrated Pollution Control, and therefore covers all plants and processes for which authorisations have been granted. The CRI could provide a useful monitoring, surveillance and analytical tool for those with an interest in environment and public health. However, further development work may be required before its full potential can be achieved.

The Royal Commission on Environmental Pollution

The Royal Commission on Environmental Pollution (RCEP) was established in 1970, "to advise on matters, both national and international, concerning the pollution of the environment, on the adequacy of research in this field, and the future possibilities of danger to the environment".[33] It has published a number of reports on topics relevant to environmental health, for example it studied transport in 1994 and soil in 1996. It might be appropriate for the government to request the RCEP to offer advice specifically on the development of EIAs to incorporate health considerations.

Health authorities and directors of public health

In April 1996 the Family Health Service Authorities and the District Health Authorities combined to form the new Health Authorities which became responsible for Family Health

Services. At the same time, changes were made to the boundaries of the health authorities in order to realign them with local authority boundaries. The new health authorities are essentially public health organisations that commission health services and work with others to improve the health of the population they serve. This involves taking account of environmental and social factors, including the potential effect of policies, programmes and projects. The core function of directors of public health (DPH) and their multidisciplinary teams has been emphasised by making the DPH one of the three statutory executive members of each health authority's management board. All health authorities are required to make arrangements to involve professionals in the full range of their work. Directors of public health are pivotal in ensuring that health professionals contribute to health authority decisions, and have a key role themselves in providing public health advice.[34] Guidance from the NHS Executive[35] confirms that the DPH's department will "act as a source of public health advice to any authority or agency whose activities impact on the health of the local population", and that the DPH "should have a role in and ensure that plans are made to respond to public health aspects of incidents relating to non-communicable environmental hazards and that his/her own role is clearly defined".

Public health doctors are employed largely by health authorities, but are increasingly advising NHS Trusts, GP fundholders, local authorities and industry. The importance of the environment within public health is increasingly in evidence in the annual reports of Directors of Public Health, some of which have concentrated entirely on this issue.[36] In order to strengthen coordination between Health Authorities and Local Authorities, the DPH annual report should include input from local authorities and contain public health indicators relevant to local government, and other agencies. In 1994 the BMA recommended that further training and education in environmental health should be available to public health doctors.[37] The need to improve training and development and career opportunities for public health professionals, as health authorities evolve as public health organisations, has also been recognised by the Chief Medical Officer.[38] Public health doctors and environmental health officers undoubtedly have an important part to play in advising on and analysing environment and health impact assessments. However, at present, the role of Health Authorities and their Directors of Public Health in the impact assessment process requires further clarification. The White Paper on the NHS[39] proposes a strategic leadership role for health authorities with the development of local Health

Improvement Programmes. In particular, a new statutory duty will be placed on health authorities to work in partnership with Local Authorities and others to identify how local action on social, environmental and economic issues will most impact on the health of local people. This will include "evaluating the health impact of local plans and developments". A study by the Chief Medical Officer is currently being undertaken to determine how the public health function can be strengthened to support this work.

Occupational health services

The development of direct legislation concerning occupational health and safety in most industrialised countries has resulted in considerable reductions in the exposure of workers to potential health hazards. In the UK, health and safety in the workplace and the environmental consequences of an organisation's activities are governed by extensive UK and EC legislation. Occupational health services work within this framework, with a primary professional responsibility to:

- promote and maintain the health, safety and welfare of people at work;
- assist in the provision at work of immediate treatment for sick and injured people;
- advise on the rehabilitation and placement in suitable work of those temporarily or permanently disabled by illness or injury;
- advise on the provision of safe and healthy conditions by informed scientific assessment of the working environment;
- educate all concerned in the attainment and preservation of good health;
- carry out or promote research into the causes of occupational diseases and injury and into the means of their prevention.

To achieve these aims, occupational physicians, nurses, administrative and other staff should be able to work as a team, and each member of the team should have clearly defined functions. The duties of a doctor in occupational medicine vary according to the occupational group involved but generally come under two distinct headings: the effects of health state on capacity for work, and the effects of work on health (see Appendix 2).

Local authorities

Local Authorities not only provide environmental health services but also have a key part to play through the planning of new development. They employ Environmental Health Officers (EHOs) who are concerned with "administration, inspection, education and regulation in respect of environmental health".[40] EHOs act as public arbiters of environmental health standards, maintaining close contact with the community, and may have a role in health education, the enforcement of environmental legislation and the provision of independent advice on environmental matters, as well as the direct maintenance of public health. In order to achieve these goals, EHOs liaise with a number of other professionals involved in the safeguard of environmental health, including public health physicians, health and safety enforcement professionals, staff of the Environment Agency, and health service workers, eg microbiologists. The Environmental Health Commission has undertaken a broad review of this subject and made recommendations for future development of environmental health in the United Kingdom.[41] The details of the review are discussed at the end of this chapter.

Local Authorities' land use development plans provide opportunities for regulating development in the interests of safeguarding health. Environmental impact assessment procedures are an important part of this. Local Authorities are uniquely placed to influence the scope of environmental assessments for new development proposals and to demand full consideration of environmental health issues. Dialogue between environmental health officers and planning officers is clearly very important.

Local Authorities also have a role in the assessment of environmental quality. For example, they are required to review and assess air quality in their locality and to establish Air Quality Management Areas (AQMAs) as part of the National Air Quality Strategy (see Appendix 3).

Non-governmental organisations and the private sector

The role of the private sector in regulating environmental hazards and people's exposure to them has become more significant in recent years.[42] In the industrial boom which followed the Second World War, few companies were aware of the environmental consequences of their activities and there was widespread failure to inform employees, customers and neighbours of any potential health hazards.[43] Since the 1960s, however, many larger companies have employed professionals who are responsible for the identification, monitoring and mitigation of potential environmental hazards. Government action to regulate industrial activity in the UK has also increased, particularly in relation to the setting of environmental quality standards, the control of environmental pollution and hazards and the authorisation of prescribed processes.

Government appointed regulators oversee the privatised electricity and gas supply industries in England, Scotland and Wales and the water services in England and Wales. These regulators have some responsibilities for environmental health, eg the Drinking Water Inspectorate checks that private water companies in England and Wales supply wholesome drinking water which complies with the requirements of the UK Regulations.

Central government lays down the statutory framework for pollution control, though many limits on emissions or discharges of pollutants are set and enforced locally. Government systems for pollution control have been influenced by the technology available and by considerations of cost, with perhaps less emphasis on desirable outcomes relating to environmental health.

As early as 1974, the concept of Best Practicable Means (BPM) was incorporated into UK legislation to control emissions to the atmosphere from particularly troublesome industries. It involves a requirement that 'the best practicable means', as judged by a

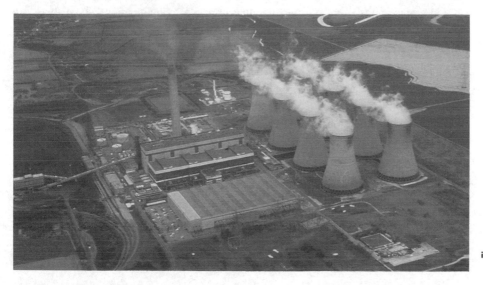

Government action to regulate industrial activity has increased since the 1960s

designated official, are utilised to address selected environmental problems. The Government's current system of Integrated Pollution Control (IPC) for industries with high pollution potential demands the use of a similar approach, ie the Best Available Techniques Not Entailing Excessive Cost (BATNEEC), to achieve the best practical environmental option. Clearly there is a risk that inferior pollution control techniques might be selected primarily on economic grounds, as the criteria for deciding what constitutes 'excessive cost' are vague. The intention is that BATNEEC should be used to direct releases to the environmental medium best able to receive them, with the objective of minimising pollution to the environment as a whole, having regard to the Best Practicable Environmental Option (BPEO). Again, an element of cost versus environmental benefit/risk is brought into play in deciding what option constitutes the BPEO. When BATNEEC standards have been set there is a risk that they will constitute a disincentive to the development of innovations which might perform even better. Most decisions have to be taken on the basis of incomplete information and sometimes in circumstances of uncertainty where there may be no technology which can plausibly be deemed to be the BATNEEC.

When the potential damage is uncertain, and yet may be significant, it is desirable and appropriate to act on the so-called 'precautionary principle'. A precautionary approach amounts to trying to be safe rather than sorry, but as O'Riordan et al have pointed out, the notion of a 'precautionary principle' has been interpreted in a variety of different ways.[44] The UK Government has used the precautionary principle to mean that "where there are significant risks of damage to the environment the government will be prepared to take precautionary action to limit the use of potentially dangerous materials or the spread of potentially dangerous pollutants, even where scientific knowledge is not conclusive, if the likely balance of costs and benefits justifies it".[45]

Companies must obtain authorisation before they can operate certain industrial processes. Processes prescribed for control under IPC have their authorisations reviewed regularly, so that in principle any developments in abatement techniques and scientific knowledge can be taken into account. The authorisation of industrial processes provides opportunities for the imposition of legally enforceable conditions, for example maximum release levels to environmental media at specific discharge points. It also provides opportunities for consultation with organisations and members of the public. However, the UK National Environmental Health Action Plan[46] does not include any specific guidance on how consultation about environmental health issues should be conducted as part of the authorisation process.

There has been a tendency for government control of environmental hazards to focus on reductions of selected and specific emissions, without addressing the wider implications. For example, the use of lead-free petrol has been encouraged, without adequate attention being paid to the desirability of not increasing exposure to benzene. That is not to say that the case against lead additives in petrol was less than compelling, but rather, that greater care should have been taken to ensure the safety of unleaded alternatives.

Effective management of health and other environmental risks requires an integrated approach which should take account of a complex set of factors which include:

- the interactions between various pollutants,
- the cumulative effects of low-level releases,
- levels of exposure (including occupational exposure) for any people in the 'receiving' environment, and
- their relative vulnerabilities to adverse effects.

Much of the motivation to manage potential environmental hazards has come from companies themselves. In the US, product-liability laws have forced the private sector to become more diligent and rigorous in identifying and avoiding suspected health hazards. The burden of accidental injuries caused by products intended for use or consumption is placed upon those who market them and is treated as a cost of production against which liability insurance can be obtained. Health injury claims have come mostly from workers exposed to hazardous substances. The application of product liability laws originated with asbestos, but has since been extended to a host of other substances.[47]

Environmental auditing has become a routine part of quality control in most large businesses who have become aware that there are potential gains in efficiency through 'environmentally sound' operations. 'Cradle to grave' management of materials and life-cycle assessments (of which an example is given in Appendix 4) can play an important part in identifying and managing potential risks to human health. Other industrial environmental management tools include economic analysis, environmental auditing and

**Table 2: Environmental management:
an overall framework[50]**

Goal	Elements	Key tools
Environmentally and economically sustainable environmental management	Human and environmental safety	• Human health risk assessment (occupational and domestic exposure). • Ecological risk assessment (plant-site and consumer releases).
	Regulatory compliance	• Manufacturing site compliance auditing. • Manufacturing site wastes reporting. • Material consumption reporting. • New chemicals testing and registration. • Product and packaging classification and labelling.
	Efficient resource use and waste management	• Manufacturing site wastes and energy consumption monitoring and reduction. • Material consumption monitoring and reduction. • Manufacturing site environmental auditing. • Supplier auditing. • Product life cycle inventory and analysis. • Eco-design. • Economic analysis.
	Addressing societal concerns	Understand: • opinion surveys. • consumer and market research. • networking. Respond: • public presentations and publications. • scientific and industry work groups. • lobbying. • reporting. • co-operation with society to find solutions to environmental problems.

Wastes = emissions to air, water and land; material consumption = raw materials consumption, both for product and packaging.

health risk assessment. However, no single tool has the capacity to include all the relevant dimensions of environmental management.

Industrial companies are uniquely placed both to reduce environmental pollution and to minimise the exposure of their own workforces to occupational hazards. But these two aspects of environmental management must be considered together. There are examples where attempts to reduce industrial releases of damaging substances have had adverse consequences for the workforce involved in implementing them. Stein[48] for example, refers to a conflict between US government agencies in the 1970s over the retro-fitting of enclosures on existing by-product coke-oven batteries to capture fugitive emissions. While the Environmental Protection Agency insisted on enclosures for compliance with air pollution regulations, the Occupational Safety and Health Administration argued against them because they created an unhealthy working environment. The technology used to reduce one adverse environmental impact can thus have significant knock-on effects on other environmental components. Reduction of pollution, for example, may be technically feasible, but very energy-expensive.

Decision-making therefore necessitates the integration of outputs from the various environmental management tools. In order to achieve this, the data must be able to be traced back to their origins, with explicit differentiation between data-based and value-laden elements, ie 'transparency'. The various management tools must also be placed within a suitable framework, not only to ensure their appropriate application, but also to enable the integration of the different outputs into a coherent form which will ultimately contribute to the goal of sustainable development. One such framework for environmental management has been developed by an international consumer goods company[49] (see Table 2). A key feature of this framework is sustainable development as a fundamental principle underpinning environmental management.

Recently there has been renewed interest in quality assurance standards both nationally and internationally. Many organisations have complied with Quality Assurance Standards ISO 9000 which ensure that they produce a reliable and safe product for their customers and clients. Following the United Nations Conference on Environment and Development (UNCED) in 1992, new Environmental Standards have been published as the ISO 14000 series. These extend the duty of quality management to the wider community and environment in which the organisation operates.[51] They are designed to cover:

environmental management systems; environmental auditing; environmental performance evaluation; environmental labelling; life-cycle assessment; and environmental aspects in product standards. ISO 14000 management system registration has become the primary requirement for doing business in many regions and industries throughout Europe. ISO 14000 series is compatible with the European Community's Eco-Management and Audit Scheme (EMAS) and British Standard 7750 which derived from the 1990 Environmental Protection Act and was reviewed and revised in January 1994. One component of the revised British Standard is an "effects register". This requires an organisation to list all the environmental effects of its activities, decide which are most significant and draw up targets for reducing these effects. The operation of these standards should provide an additional method of assessing the capability of a project proponent to protect human health as part of their proposed development plans. The Department of Trade and Industry and the Department of the Environment, Transport and the Regions should consider how these quality standards can be applied more formally to the impact assessment process in the UK.

European action

Growing international concern about the environment, human health and interactions between them has promoted a number of collaborative initiatives intended to address human health issues. In 1984, for example, the Member States of the World Health Organisation (WHO) in the European Region set up a *Health for All* (HFA) strategy with targets to be met by the year 2000. These targets, updated in 1991, include eight which relate specifically to environmental health. The first European Conference on Environment and Health was held in Frankfurt in 1989. A European Charter on Environment and Health extended the HFA strategy with respect to the environment and was unanimously approved.

However, until the Treaty on European Union (Treaty of Maastricht) was ratified in 1993, there was no direct legal basis for an EU health policy.[52] Paragraph 1 of Article 129 of the Maastricht Treaty states that:

"The Community shall contribute towards ensuring a high level of human health protection by encouraging cooperation between Member States and, if necessary, lending support to their action.

Community action shall be directed towards the prevention of diseases, in particular the major health scourges, including drug dependence, by promoting research into their causes and their transmission, as well as health information and education. Health protection requirements shall form a constituent part of the Community's other policies."

The European Commission has issued clarification that Article 129 "requires the Commission to check that proposals for policies, and implementing measures and instruments, do not have an adverse impact on health, or create conditions which undermine the promotion of health".[53] However, despite this commitment to prospective health impact assessment there is, at present, no systematic means to its implementation. This situation requires correction, particularly in relation to the health impact of EU policies such as the funding of tobacco production and the promotion of whole fat dairy produce.[54]

The Second European Conference on Environment and Health was held in Helsinki in 1994. The WHO Regional Office for Europe produced an environmental health action plan for Europe (EHAPE) which has now been finalised and published. This sets out a blueprint for the preparation of national environmental health action plans (NEHAPs) as well as a Europe-wide plan. At the Helsinki conference, European member states endorsed a Declaration committing their respective health and environment departments to the joint development of "action plans on health and the environment"... which "should be integrated in or closely linked with both environmental action programmes and with health planning processes". The close integration of environmental and health issues was also identified as "an important step towards sustainability".[55] The UK's National Environmental Health Action Plan was published in 1996 and is discussed in detail below.

UK National Environmental Health Action Plan

The focus of the UK National Environmental Health Action Plan (NEHAP)[56] is the surveillance and study of existing environments and environmental health problems, including hazard identification and risk assessment. There are also implicit references to the need for health impact assessment. These include a statement of objectives for an institutional framework as follows:

"To ensure, through the establishment of appropriate government machinery, that decisions and long-term strategic planning affecting the natural environment, and through it health, are taken not merely on the basis of economic factors alone but also with full consideration of potential environmental health consequences, in accordance with the requirements of sustainable development".

It is also stated that "the government will continue to ... assess the impact of ... hazards ... arising from proposed environmental development or change upon the health of the general public or of vulnerable groups".

There is a brief mention of the Department of Health's 1995 document entitled *Policy Appraisal and Health*[57] (which will be discussed in greater detail in Chapter 6) but the main thrust of that paper is not integrated into the report. There is also a brief mention of environmental health impact assessments in the section on new investments in energy suggesting that pollution controls and environmental impact assessments provide effective means with which environmental health impacts can be regulated, but that suggestion is not substantiated.

Environmental Health Commission: *Agendas for Change*

In 1996 the Chartered Institute of Environmental Health established a Commission to undertake a broad review of environmental health and to make recommendations for its future development in the United Kingdom.[58] The Commission acknowledged that health and the environment have always been intimately related. Bad environments can be a cause of ill health, even mortality. Good environments contribute directly to quality of life and well being. In recent years, however, the subjects have tended to drift apart, both conceptually and in institutional policies. Health policy, resources and institutions have concentrated mainly on care and treatment of the sick, whilst at the same time, environmental policy has broadened its range, and has sometimes given insufficient priority to health-related objectives. This 'drifting apart' of public and environmental health needs to be reversed locally, nationally and internationally. Improvements require the reintegration of environment and health policies and organisations, and the integration of environmental health objectives within a broader strategic framework of sustainable development.

The Commission made a number of recommendations beginning with action needed at local level. These recommendations included:

- the need for local authorities to involve local communities, health authorities and other relevant bodies from the public, private and voluntary sectors, in preparing their strategies;
- the possible re-siting of public health medicine, and health promotion specialties from the NHS to local government;
- the preparation by local authorities of an annual public report on the health of the local population covering all aspects of local government which affect health. This should include the routine collection and analysis of health and environmental quality data providing the basis for action; and importantly,
- a requirement for local authorities, in collaboration with other bodies, to develop techniques for integrated environmental health impact assessment.

At a national level, the Commission recommended that:

- key government departments should establish a joint unit to co-ordinate the development of an integrated approach to policy on environment, health and sustainable development. This unit should lead an initiative to establish and co-ordinate a coherent national research programme for environment, health and sustainable development issues.

The report provides a good starting point for debate, which can be expected to lead to beneficial reform and long-term improvements in environmental health.

Planning of new development

The Town and Country Planning Act of 1947 remains the foundation of the present planning system, in theory providing the opportunity to manage new developments in the interests of public environmental health.

Options for planning to safeguard environmental health are provided by two main mechanisms: the production of local development plans and environmental impact assessment (EIA). The former provides scope for looking forward and taking account of the overall needs of the public in zoning for new development. EIA, on the other hand, permits detailed assessment of the potential environmental health implications of proposed new developments and is the focus of this report.

In the UK, planning decisions are made by local planning authorities (LPAs).[59] The LPA is required to take EIAs into account together with other factors. It has been established that EIAs do not usually contain substantial discussions about human health issues[60] (see Appendix 1). However, it is possible that health impact assessments are submitted to the LPA from some other source. No survey of planning decisions has yet been carried out in this regard.

Planning decisions are published in a register maintained by each LPA and if planning permission is refused, reasons must be given. The project proponent has a right of appeal. Appeals are heard centrally at planning inquiries conducted by the Planning Inspectorate. The outcome of all planning appeals is held in a database, currently containing about 46,500 items. A search of this database has revealed 46 cases (0.1%) in which human health hazards were explicitly mentioned. Thirty-one of these were allowed to proceed and 15 were refused. About half of the 46 cases involved incinerator plants and the remainder covered a diverse range of projects. The major perceived health hazards in the 46 appeals were traffic injuries, noise and dust, low frequency electromagnetic radiation from power lines, pollution of aquifers, chemical plant explosion and hazardous waste disposal in landfill sites. Further analysis is required to determine how the perceived health hazards affect the outcome of the planning inquiry.

3

Environmental impact assessment: development and current UK provision

Introduction

Worldwide, mechanisms for fully integrated action on environmental and health issues are quite limited. In the UK, for example, it has been found that while legislation gives scope for coverage of human health issues, this is not regarded as a priority by most public authorities (see Appendix 6). With respect to the development of new urban and industrial infrastructure and the introduction of new government policies and plans, however, environmental impact assessments (EIAs) provide an obvious way forward. Not only have EIAs been implemented through legislation throughout the world, but they require a complex, integrated and cross-sectoral analysis of the effects on numerous aspects of the environment. Furthermore, considerable progress has already been made in some countries in formally integrating health impact assessments into EIAs (see Appendix 5).

Environmental impact assessment

The UK Department of Environment (now Department of the Environment, Transport and the Regions) has defined EIA as a "technique and a process by which information about the environmental effects of a 'project' is collected, both by the developer and from other sources, and taken into account by the planning authority in forming their judgements on whether the development should go ahead".[1]

'**Projects**' refers to development actions and are divided into two main categories or Schedules by the UK Town and Country Planning (Assessment of Environmental Effects) Regulations 1988.*

Schedule 1 projects (referred to in Annex I of EC Directive 85/337/EEC) include:
- Crude oil refineries
- Thermal power stations, nuclear power stations and other nuclear reactors
- Installations for the permanent storage or disposal of radioactive waste
- Integrated works for the initial melting of cast-iron or steel
- Installations for the extraction, processing, and transformation of asbestos
- Integrated chemical installations
- Construction of motorways, express roads, long-distance railway lines and airports
- Waste disposal installations for the incineration, chemical treatment or landfill of toxic or dangerous waste, etc.

Schedule 2 projects (Annex II) include:
- Agricultural projects, eg restructuring rural land holdings; use of uncultivated land or semi-natural areas for intensive agricultural purposes etc
- Extractive industry projects, eg deep drillings, peat or mineral extraction, underground or open-cast mining etc
- Energy industry, eg industrial installations for the production of electricity (not covered under Schedule 1 above); installations for carrying gas, steam or hot water; transmission of electrical energy by overhead cables etc
- Process metals, eg iron and steelworks, boiler making, manufacture and assembly of motor vehicles or aircraft etc
- Manufacture of glass
- Chemical industry
- Food manufacture
- Textile, leather, wood and paper industries
- Rubber industry
- Infrastructure projects, eg industrial-estate development
- Other projects, eg holiday villages, hotel complexes, racing and test tracks for cars and motorcycles, waste water treatment plants etc.

These categories may change as a result of the implementation of the new EIA Directive[2] in the UK. Member States must comply with the Directive by 14 March 1999

In setting out formal procedures for the assessment of different categories of environmental impact, EIAs potentially provide a mechanism for effectively considering the relationships between proposed new developments and human and environmental health.

EIA is a predictive tool employed before the implementation of a project which, when applied appropriately and effectively, is an important and integral part of the planning of a project that should reduce, mitigate or ameliorate adverse environmental effects of that project. A key characteristic of any EIA should be the participation of, and consultation with, affected parties. The extent, nature and constituencies of participation will, however, vary between countries and the relevant planning systems laid down by law or regulatory authority guidance.

Environmental impact assessment (EIA) is a technique and a process by which information about the environmental effects of a project is collected, both by the developer and from other sources, and taken into account by the planning authority in forming their judgements on whether the development should go ahead.[3] The UK must carry out EIAs in order to comply with the European Directive,[4] and its subsequent amendment.[5]

As there are many diverse systems for EIA in use throughout the world, no single approach can capture the full range of alternative methods. Nevertheless, EIA processes do tend to share common elements and stages and these are illustrated in Figure 1. It should be noted however that not all the elements shown in Figure 1 are legal requirements within every EIA system, eg scoping and project monitoring. Ideally, the EIA process should be interactive, including scope for feedback from later stages so that the project proposal can be modified to incorporate the findings from the provisional assessment. Similarly, the terms of reference of an EIA should be flexible enough to allow modification to take account of the results of public consultation.

EIA is normally wider in scope and less quantitative than some other techniques, such as cost-benefit analysis (which will be discussed in Chapter 5). EIAs encompass a wide range of disciplines which have evolved to deal with different types of human activity and different categories of environmental impacts. The academic literature refers, for example, to social impact assessments, fiscal impact assessments, demographic impact assessments, ecological impact assessments and health impact assessments.[6] EIAs have proved a valuable tool to aid decision-making partly because they provide analytical frameworks for considering a range of different kinds of impacts and their interactions. EIAs can help to clarify some of the different trade-offs associated with a proposed development action, without necessarily identifying any uniquely optimal solution.[7]

Figure 1: A generic EIA process

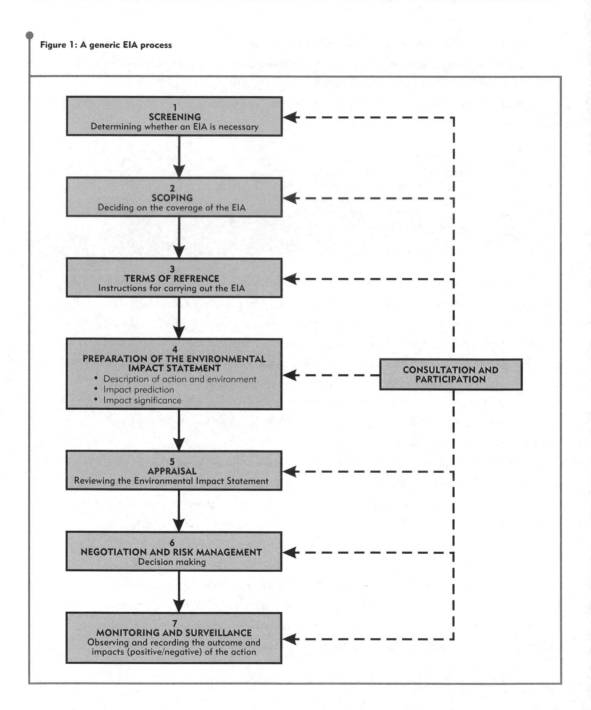

Strategic environmental assessment

The process of EIA can be applied specifically to individual development projects or, more strategically, to proposed policies, plans and programmes, when the process is referred to as strategic environmental assessment (SEA).

Strategic environmental assessment (SEA) can be defined as "the formalised, systematic and comprehensive process of evaluating the environmental impacts of a policy, plan or programme and its alternatives, including the preparation of a written report on the findings of that evaluation, and using the findings in publicly accountable decision-making".[8] SEAs are not mandatory in the UK at present, although a draft EC Directive[9] is under consideration.

Strategic decision-making stages offer a much better opportunity to address cumulative impacts of numerous individual projects, linkages to other policies, and sustainability issues than project-based EIA. SEA therefore has a vital part to play in safeguarding environmental and human health. The role of SEA in relation to the health impact assessment of policies, programmes and plans is considered later; however, potential benefits and rationale of SEA are that it:

- promotes integrated environment and development decision-making;
- facilitates the design of environmentally-sustainable policies and plans;
- provides for consideration of a larger range of alternatives than is normally possible in project EIA;
- takes account, where possible, of cumulative effects and global change;
- strengthens and streamlines project EIA by prior identification of impacts and information requirements, clearance of strategic issues and concerns, and reduces time and effort taken to conduct reviews.[10]

In some countries and federal jurisdictions, SEA provision and practice is at an equivalent level, eg Denmark, Hong Kong, Western Australia. Other countries have recently established or are introducing SEA systems, eg Norway and Austria. Many developing countries have SEA-type provisions, eg regional assessment in China, and central and eastern European countries in transition, have strong planning traditions on which SEA could be built. In the UK, SEA is not mandatory at present. Instead, there is a framework of guidance by the Government on environmental appraisal of national policies and development plans, such as *Policy Appraisal and the Environment*, which is discussed in Chapter 5. A draft EC Directive[11] is under consideration which provides the UK with an opportunity to influence the development of an SEA system which will take account of existing UK practice in environmental appraisal of policies and plans. There is a need to explicitly link SEA to the aims of sustainable development, but at the present time, the relationship between SEA and other environmental management processes and policy evaluation tools needs clarification.

Social impact assessment

Environmental impact assessments (EIAs) have clearly been formulated with the physical rather than the social environment in mind, where the emphasis is on conservation of nature, ecology, sustainability, traffic, air pollution and climate etc. Social impacts are often underestimated and assessment is lacking in methodology and practice.[12] In some countries social impact assessment is regarded as a separate process, whereas in others it may form part of, or be carried out in parallel to, EIAs or HIAs.[13] Gilpin has defined social impact assessment as "an assessment of the impact on people and society of major policies, plans, programmes, activities, and developments".[14] Social impacts or effects are those changes in social relations between members of a community, society and institution, resulting from external change. The changes might be physical or psychological, involving social cohesion, general lifestyle, cultural life, attitudes and values, social tranquillity, relocation of residents, and severance or separation and can be both positive or negative.[15]

Where social impacts are included in the assessment they are often presented as a list of factors and isolated symptoms. Social impact assessment needs to be further developed and integrated to consider the system of inter-relationships between these factors. A computer-based modelling technique for conducting such an SIA has been developed at the Bartlett Graduate School. It provides a framework of analysis of the built environment and all forms of social and economic activity patterns and inter-relationships between them. The analysis of patterns is based on concrete data and empirical observation and thus provides a systematic prediction model for potential impacts on proposed designs.[16]

It is important to note that social impacts can be both negative and positive. For example, a series of reports, based on the Sizewell B Public Inquiry, were produced as a result of monitoring and auditing of the local socio-economic impacts of the nuclear power station construction project. Although the predictions were not formally packaged as an EIS, research was extensive and comprehensive.[17] Findings from the survey of local residents carried out during the construction period revealed increased traffic and work disruption as major negative impacts. The main positive impacts of the project were seen to be increased employment, additional trade and ameliorative measures associated with it.

Unfortunately, to date, social impact assessment is frequently only poorly dealt with in impact assessments.[18] In 1995, the BMA commented that although there is a need for further research, there is currently sufficient evidence available to enable health, including social implications, to be taken into account in developing effective policy in areas such as environment, housing and transport.[19] Such data should be drawn upon in the health and social impact assessment of new developments, policies and plans in these areas. An enhanced social environmental impact assessment could be a valuable tool for the development of plans and design proposals, providing local authorities with a constructive framework of environmental assessment within which to involve the affected community/statutory bodies.[20]

Health impact assessment

Health impact assessment (HIA) is defined in this report as a methodology which enables the identification, prediction and evaluation of the likely changes in health risk, both positive and negative, (single or collective), of a policy, programme, plan or development action on a defined population. These changes may be direct and immediate, or indirect and delayed. In 1946, the World Health Organisation defined human health as "a complete state of physical, mental and social well-being and not merely the absence of disease or infirmity".[21] One consequence of the WHO definition is that there are stronger, but largely unexplored, linkages between health impact assessment and social impact

> **Health impact assessment** (HIA) is a methodology which aims to identify, predict and evaluate the likely changes in health risk, both positive and negative (single or collective), of a policy, programme, plan, or development action on a defined population. Ideally, health impact assessments should always include consideration of physical, mental and social impacts.

assessment. Ideally, health impact assessments should always include consideration of physical, mental and social impacts, as well as potential diseases.

To be effective, HIA must provide a mechanism for identifying the full spectrum of potential 'health hazards', evaluating their potential for causing harm and assessing their risk of occurrence to any particular group/target at any particular time/place. The ultimate aim is informed 'health risk management'.[22] The output of an HIA (usually a report) will be presented to decision-makers/planning authorities who must then evaluate the relative importance of the impacts that have been identified in a wider context. However, it is important to remember that decision-makers may not be medical or health specialists, and so the report should always include a summary in non-technical language to enable comparison of impacts by decision-makers and allow members of the general public to gain an appreciation of the issues involved.

Unlike EIAs, HIAs do not exist as a separate procedure within the UK. The implementation of an HIA as a distinct activity has usually been under the provisions of an EIA and related legislation. However, a review of ten UK environmental impact statements (EISs) produced to summarise the results of EIAs concluded that negligible attention had been paid to human health.[23] A further review commissioned by the BMA for this present report similarly found that human health issues are not regarded as a priority and health did not feature to any significant extent in the 39 EISs reviewed (see Appendix 6).

The 39 environmental impact statements (EISs) for proposed developments in the UK were selected at random from a collection held by Oxford Brookes University, and were reviewed to establish the extent and depth of impacts on human health. The EISs were all produced between 1988 and 1994 and included proposals for clinical waste incinerators, landfill sites, opencast coal mines, road improvements and bypasses, sewage treatment works, power stations and agricultural units. The potential magnitude and severity of the potential impacts on human beings and their health of those proposals varied between the different types of developments and between individual projects of the same broad type.

The majority of the EISs (72%) did not list in their tables of contents nor discuss explicitly in the document, human health or health-related issues. 13% of the EISs provided sections concerned with 'impacts on human beings and/or local communities' but they were not specifically related to health, while sections on 'safety' and/or 'hazards' were included in 15% of the EISs. Only one EIS out of the sample of 39 included a section which made direct reference to human health. It is appropriate that HIAs should be considered as a component of EIAs, rather than as separate and parallel activities, because of the importance of developing an integrated approach to health and the environment. In addition, the planning machinery necessary for impact assessments has already evolved and it would be inefficient to attempt to duplicate or replace it.

The value of EIAs for effective environmental planning and management is now widely recognised and EIAs in some form are required by law in over half the countries of the world. Since the UK implemented an EC Directive in 1988, EIAs have become regular and required elements in important planning procedures.

European EIA and SEA legislation

EIA

The European Commission (EC) passed a Council Directive (85/337/EEC) on 27 June 1985 on 'the assessment of the effects of certain public and private projects on the environment'. The EIA Directive was intended to ensure that any public or private project likely to have significant effects on the environment is subject to systematic assessment of these effects before development consent is given.[24] This was subsequently amended in 1997 by Council Directive (97/11/EC),[25] which tightened and extended many of the provisions of the original Directive, particularly with regard to screening to determine whether or not projects should be subject to an EIA.

Member States were given three years to implement the first EIA Directive,[26] either by integrating EIAs into existing development consent procedures, or by creating entirely new procedures. The UK opted to implement the Directive through various sets of regulations which supplemented the pre-existing planning system: in particular the Town and Country Planning (Assessment of Environmental Effects) Regulations 1988 (SI No.

1199). Procedures for carrying out EIAs in the UK are outlined in a guide published by the Department of the Environment, Transport and the Regions (DETR) and the Welsh Office.[27] There are many other regulations which have included the requirements of the EC Directive, including the Highways Act 1980, Section 105A of which deals with EIAs for proposed new motorways and trunk roads in England and Wales. Similar provisions are found in Sections 20A and 55A of the Roads (Scotland) Act 1984 and Article 39B of the Roads (Northern Ireland) Order 1980. Technical guidance dealing with the practical issues of EIAs is dealt with in the *Design Manual for Roads and Bridges* (Volume 11).[28] Further regulations and technical guidance will be required to cover the requirements of the new EIA Directive[29] prior to its implementation in March 1999. In July 1997 Government issued a consultation paper setting out the general principles which will underpin the Government's proposals for implementation of the new Directive.[30] A second consultation paper issued in December 1997[31] sets out more detailed proposals for refining the way in which the need for EIA is determined in the UK. Specific aspects of the Government proposals are discussed at relevant points throughout this report. The Government plans to undertake further separate consultations during 1998 on each set of proposed regulations necessary to implement the Directive in the UK.

SEA

The EIA Directive is still based on a relatively restricted definition of an EIA, requiring it only for individual projects ('project EIA'). However, there is increasing pressure for EIAs to be applied at higher tiers in the planning process. The application of EIA to policies, plans, and programmes is known as 'strategic environmental assessment' (or SEA). SEA makes it possible to complement 'policy and need' inquiries with the more site-specific inquiries normally carried out at the project level. SEA can also provide frameworks within which wider issues of natural resource conservation and sustainability can be addressed.

Plans for a Directive on SEA were first expressed by the European Commission in the early 1980s. At that time it was considered that this would cover policies, plans and programmes. Following a period of research, the circulation of a series of draft SEA directives began in 1991. However, during this consultation period, the coverage of policies was deleted. The present draft of the European Directive on SEA[32] requires formal assessment of the environmental implications of new or modified plans and programmes which are adopted as part of the town and country planning decision-making process for the purpose of establishing the framework for subsequent development consents. These include strategic plans and programmes adopted in the energy, waste, water, industry, telecommunication and tourism sectors, and certain transport infrastructure plans and programmes.

There are many similarities between the proposed SEA Directive and the EIA Directive on which it is modelled, including requirements for screening, scoping and the preparation of an environmental statement. The SEA Directive should enable the consideration of alternative development options in a holistic way. An important aspect of the proposal is that it will allow the assessment of the cumulative impacts of numerous, individual projects which are undertaken as part of a larger scale plan or programme. However, the opportunity, provided by the SEA Directive, to implement effective monitoring and data collection programmes may be missed. There is currently no provision for monitoring of environmental effects of plans and programmes following implementation. The scope of the SEA Directive, like its EIA counterpart, only requires the assessment of the "significant direct and indirect effects ... on human beings".[33] There is no specific provision or guidance for assessing the effects on human health. There may be problems with the implementation of the SEA Directive across the entire EU, because Member States use different planning systems and adoption procedures. If provision for assessment of policies was reinstated, the SEA Directive could catalyse the development of an integrated approach to the health and environmental impact assessment of policies, programmes and plans across Europe.

UK regulations

The UK Town and Country Planning (Assessment of Environmental Effects) Regulations 1998 divide projects into two main categories or Schedules (reproduced from the Annexes in the EIA Directive).[34] Schedule 1 lists projects (including nuclear power stations, for example) which automatically require an EIA due to the significance of their potential impacts on the environment. The number of projects in this category has been increased by the new EIA Directive[35] and now includes radioactive waste reprocessing plants, waste incinerators (of over 100 tonnes per day capacity) and overhead powerlines (over 15 km in length), for example. Schedule 2 projects require EIAs in some circumstances, depending on factors such as their size and location. In the UK, the planning authorities have an important role in determining when EIAs are deemed necessary for such projects.

The Regulations were amended in 1994,[36] to clarify the circumstances under which EIAs should be required for Schedule 2 projects (Annex II in the EIA Directive). Those amendments increased the range of projects subject to EIAs and required improved measures for dealing with potential trans-boundary effects, such as those associated with the long-distance transfer of atmospheric pollutants, ie across country borders. As part of the proposals for the implementation of the new EC Directive,[37] the UK Government plans to revise its existing guidance to help planning authorities decide whether a project is likely to require an EIA.[38]

Where an EIA is required, the EIA Directive[39] specifies the minimum information which should be provided to the planning authorities concerned with the project and its likely effects in the form of an environmental impact statement (EIS). The statutory provisions of the UK Regulations are set out in Schedule 3 to the Town and Country Planning (Assessment of Environmental Effects) Regulations 1988 and the Highways Act 1980 (Schemes and Orders). In summary, the environmental impact statement prepared for the EIA must include specified information as follows:

- a description of the development proposed, comprising information about the site and the design and size or scale of the development;
- the data necessary to identify and assess the main effects which that development is likely to have on the environment;
- a description of the likely significant effects, direct and indirect, on the environment of the development, explained by reference to its possible impact on: human beings; flora; fauna; soil; water; air; climate; the landscape; the interaction between any of the foregoing; material assets, and the cultural heritage;
- where significant adverse effects are identified with respect to any of the foregoing, a description of the measures envisaged in order to avoid, reduce or remedy those effects; and
- a summary in non-technical language of the information specified above.

The EIA Directive, and consequently the UK Regulations, does not explicitly require the assessment of impacts on human health. Unfortunately, this weakness has not been corrected by the new EIA Directive.[40] Instead 'human beings' are listed as an environmental 'factor' for which significant adverse effects must be assessed. Development proponents are also required to address any relevant interactions between human beings and other components of the environment, such as the soil, water and air. Given that there are a number of environmental effects which may find expression in adverse impacts on human health (for example, pollution of drinking water or air), some form of HIA is clearly appropriate. It can also be argued that an HIA would often be necessary to fulfil the requirements of the Directive in any case where 'significant adverse effects' can be demonstrated. However, unless in implementing the new EIA Directives the UK Government acts to take advantage of the clause that "Member States may lay down stricter rules to protect the environment",[41] in order to explicitly include health, the shortcomings of the present EIA process are likely to be perpetuated.

DETR guide to environmental impact assessment procedures

The Department of the Environment, Transport and the Regions' guide to EIA procedures[42] includes a checklist of "matters to be considered for inclusion in an environmental statement" which makes no specific reference to the need for assessment of potential impacts on human health *per se*.

Appendix 4 of the guide suggests that "information describing the project" should include details of "residues and emissions", while a subsequent section on information "describing the site and its environment" suggests that "population-proximity and numbers" should be specified. This requirement is listed rather obscurely under the 'physical features'. However, the subsequent guidance on the 'assessment of effects' does not indicate that it might be appropriate to consider the relationship between residues, emissions and the health of the population. It refers only to the need to consider changes in the size of the population arising from the development and any consequential environmental effects. Similarly, reference is made to the effects of pollutants on water and air quality and to the need to consider "secondary effects resulting from the interaction of separate effects", but again, there is no specific reference to the need to consider the potential implications of pollution on human health.

Other sources of advice, for example the Highways Agency *Design Manual for Roads and Bridges*,[43] similarly make no specific reference to the need for assessment of potential impacts on human health. However, the Highways Agency recommended that impacts on some environmental media should be evaluated against national and international quality standards. Some of these, for example air quality standards,[44] are determined by reference to human health (see Appendix 3).

Risk of major incidents/accidents

Risk of accidents is the subject of separate European legislation and is therefore not covered explicitly by the European Directive on EIA or the UK Regulations.[45] However, the DETR

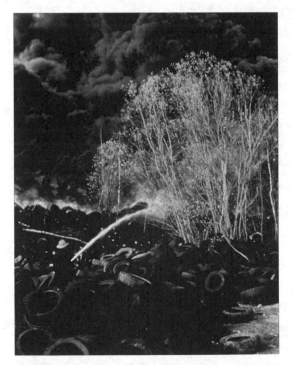

guide to EIA procedures suggests that it is appropriate to indicate the preventative measures which would be taken in the event of a major accident following development involving "materials that could be harmful to the environment (including people)". Where a development involves such materials, it may be appropriate to indicate compliance with the Health and Safety at Work etc Act 1974 "and its relevant statutory provisions such as the Control of Industrial Major Accident Hazards Regulations 1984". The guide also emphasises the desirability of considering the risk of accidents and the general environmental effects of developments together.

The Highways Agency makes an assessment of the risk of accidents to users of major highways. Their guidance also contains a procedure for assessing the risk of accidental

An EIA should consider the risk of major accident together with the general environmental effects of a development

spillages on the highway, but no assessment is made of any consequential health risk. The Environment Agency has published an initial assessment of the environmental impact of road transport which considers issues such as accidents which cause pollution.[46] But again, human health is not explicitly addressed. A more in-depth study is planned which will seek to quantify the risks, and assess the relative merits of options to prevent environmental damage, and to determine the economic impact of these measures.

Other relevant legislation

While legislation for EIAs in the UK has provided scope for controlling the effects of proposed new development on human health, other legislation has a role in regulating some of the impacts of development which may have implications for health. These include: Health and Safety at Work etc Act 1974, Control of Industrial Major Accident Hazards Regulations 1984, Environment Act 1995. It is important that the relationships between different pieces of environmental legislation should be considered in relation to the effectiveness with which existing and potential new impacts on human health are regulated.

Conclusion

There is an urgent need to revise the requirements for the inclusion of health in the EIA process, and for the development of appropriate methodology for conducting health impact assessments. This will be difficult and complex, for a variety of reasons. Some difficulties are a consequence of the complexity of the relationships between human and environmental health. For example, where pollution is concerned, it can be very difficult to extrapolate the results of laboratory-based toxicological tests, carried out on experimental animals, to people. Estimating effects at the population level is particularly difficult, as actual levels of exposure (especially locally) are difficult to measure or predict.

One of the main difficulties in incorporating human health more directly has been the general lack of dialogue between those in the health care professions and those concerned with environmental regulation. The establishment of this dialogue will be important to ensure that the consequences of new developments for human health are acceptable, and that human health is properly safeguarded by environmental regulation.

Good examples can be found where effective, integrated assessments of environmental and human health impacts have been carried out. Some of them are given in this report. By building health impact assessment (HIA) into the EIA process it should be possible to ensure that the relationships between human health and the biophysical environment are taken into account in the planning of new developments. It will become clear during the course of this report, that the effectiveness of impact assessment depends on its earliest possible integration into the planning and design of new urban and industrial infrastructure. Increasingly, it is becoming clear that HIA will have to be applied strategically to ensure that the cross-sectoral implications of development can be considered, and that the effects of policies, programmes and plans on human health are properly addressed.

CHAPTER 4

The inclusion of human health in the environmental impact assessment process

Introduction

During its development throughout the world, environmental impact assessment (EIA) has become steadily broader and more integrative.[1] However, failure to fully integrate, or even to give attention to, the relationships between the biophysical environment and human health remains a major deficiency in a number of countries, including the UK. Although the existing legislation for EIA in the UK provides scope for controlling the effects of proposed new developments on human health, its potential has not been realised. This has been clearly illustrated through a review commissioned by the BMA to examine coverage of impacts on human health in 39 environmental impact statements (see Appendix 6). The review examined a range of environmental impact statements for the level of coverage of human health issues. It was estimated that potential health effects had received adequate coverage in approximately 28% only of the statements studied. Although legislation gives scope for coverage of human environmental health issues, this was clearly not seen as a priority by developers or consultants. More importantly, the statements examined failed to provide the information necessary to assess the likely implications of new developments for human health, and the populations likely to be affected by developments were rarely identified.

A number of possible explanations have been suggested for the lack of emphasis given to issues of environmental health and safety in environmental impact assessments:

- the statements reviewed were for developments unlikely to have significant impacts on health;

- proponents wish to downplay potential impacts on health;

- human health impact assessment is complex and would incur additional costs;

- legislation fails to make human health impact assessment an explicit requirement;

- there are no clear procedures or methodologies for assessing the health implications of new developments.

Although the evidence obtained did not make it possible to determine which of these explanations is most likely, the information is still of assistance in considering ways of improving upon the current inadequate situation.

Incorporating HIA with EIA

In order to achieve an integrated approach, health impact assessment needs to be built more explicitly into the machinery of development planning in the UK. This would ensure that the individual and collective effects of development on human health are taken into account in its planning and regulation. Health impact assessment should thus be considered a component of EIA, not a separate and parallel activity. The planning machinery for environmental impact assessment is already in place and it would be inappropriate to duplicate or replace it. This report considers how the processes of health impact assessment and environmental impact assessment (EIA) might be integrated.

For terminological convenience the report refers primarily to 'projects' (and EIA) although policies, programmes and plans are included except where otherwise stated. The latter three fall into the category of strategic environmental assessment, which is similar to the EIA process on which it is based. The examples contained in this report, therefore, relate to project-level and strategic-level health impact assessment.

The way in which health and the expertise of health specialists can be included in each of the stages of the EIA process is illustrated in Figure 2. Each of the stages of the EIA process is discussed below in relation to health. Note that the EIA process is cyclic and the

addition, lack of awareness of health hazards and risks can contribute to failure of the planning authorities to require the assessment of health impacts for a proposal.

DoE Circular 15/88 (Welsh Office Circular 23/88)[8] includes some general guidance as to how 'significance' should be assessed in determining the need for EIAs with respect to Schedule 2 projects. In summary, it suggests that the following three criteria should be applied, with the need for EIAs depending on:

- whether the project is of more than local importance, principally in terms of physical scale;
- whether the project is intended for a particularly sensitive location, for example a national park or a site of special scientific interest, and for that reason may have significant effects on the area's environment even though the project is not on a major scale;
- whether the project is thought likely to give rise to particularly complex or adverse effects, for example in terms of the discharge of pollutants.

This guidance can be used by planning authorities in determining the need for EIAs with respect to general environmental concerns. No specific guidance is given concerning the potential significance of human health impacts, but further indicative criteria, summarised in an appendix of the DoE Circular,[9] do make reference to the importance of proximity to centres of population. For example, industrial estate developments may require an EIA where "there are significant numbers of dwellings in close proximity to the site of the proposed estate". Despite the requirements to undertake EIA only where the above criteria apply, the Highways Agency operates a policy whereby it undertakes EIA for all its motorway and trunk road schemes in the National Trunk Road Programme.

In order to meet the requirements to implement the new EIA Directive in the UK by the year 1999, the Government proposes to revise its existing guidance,[10,11,12] to planning authorities. The revised guidance will take account of new project types which have been added to Annex II, such as golf courses, shopping centres and car parks and the new Annex III to the Directive which specifies the selection criteria to be taken into account in assessing whether a project requires EIA.[13] The Annex III selection criteria include project characteristics (eg size, waste production, nuisance and risk of accidents), location of projects (eg in densely populated areas) and characteristics of potential impacts (eg size of affected population or geographical area, duration, frequency and reversibility of impacts). There are three main types of project identified by the Government as being likely to give rise to significant environmental effects:

- projects of more than local importance, principally in terms of physical scale;
- smaller projects which are proposed for particularly sensitive or vulnerable locations, eg Sites of Special Scientific Interest; and
- projects with unusually complex and potentially adverse environmental effects (eg in terms of discharge of pollutants).

The Government proposes to set 'indicative' thresholds for these three types of project to give further guidance on when an EIA may be required. However, in order to focus resources on projects which could have significant effects, 'exclusive' thresholds will also be set, below which there will be a clear presumption that EIA is not required. Projects above this threshold will then be considered on a case-by-case basis. The Secretary of State (or the Department of the Environment in Northern Ireland) may, however, exercise the power to require an EIA, even if it falls below the exclusive threshold (see Figure 3).

Although thresholds such as close proximity to houses, schools, hospitals and the risk of significant urbanising effects have been identified by the Government as factors which *may* indicate that a project requires EIA, the consultation document[14] makes no explicit reference to the need to screen projects for potential risks to human health. Clearly, the process by which projects are screened to determine the need for an EIA needs to be adjusted so that potential significant impacts on human health are included more explicitly. In order to do this, a systematic review of the health hazards associated with developments in each sector should be carried out to produce a checklist that can be used during the screening process to guide the planning authority and developers as to whether a project is likely to have significant human health impact. This will facilitate the inclusion of the first step:

A
Identification
of health hazards
(and benefits)
associated with the
project

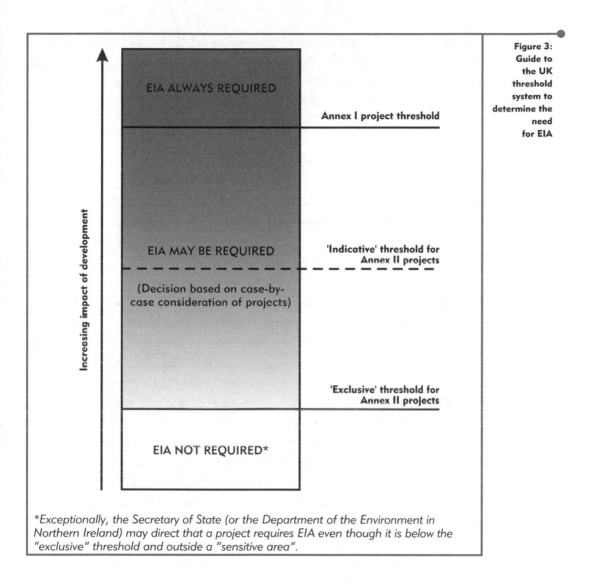

Figure 3: Guide to the UK threshold system to determine the need for EIA

Exceptionally, the Secretary of State (or the Department of the Environment in Northern Ireland) may direct that a project requires EIA even though it is below the "exclusive" threshold and outside a "sensitive area".

Hazards both directly and indirectly associated with the development should be included in the checklist. The importance of each should be determined according to its frequency and severity. Other determinants may be sociological or political. The list should include perceived hazards for which there is little or no evidence but high public concern. Severity is a subjective concept. For example, the incidence of Cruetzfeldt-Jakob Disease in the UK is about 0.5 per million (40-50 cases)[15] however, the incidence of lung cancer is much higher, approximately 56.8 per hundred thousand for men and 29.9 per hundred thousand for women in 1993.[16] Often there is more public concern about exposure to less frequent hazards, especially those which are beyond the control of the people who may be vulnerable to those hazards.

2.   Scoping

Once a decision has been taken (via the screening process) that an EIA is required for a proposal, it is necessary to determine the scope of the EIA and to draw up suitable terms of reference. Scoping procedures are used to determine the range of issues which should be addressed in the EIA and to identify those which should be studied in detail. In some countries, eg USA, scoping studies are a formal requirement and are standardised. In the UK, scoping is not a legally mandated step. The original draft of the new EIA Directive[17] proposed that scoping should be mandatory; however, this recommendation did not appear in the final Directive. It was replaced with the provisions that "if the developer so requests ... the competent authority shall give an opinion on the information to be supplied by the developer" as part of the assessment. "Member States may require the competent authority to give such an opinion irrespective of whether the developer so requests". Changes in UK legislation due to take effect in 1999[18] mean that local planning offices, if requested, will advise a developer, or those making the assessment of his proposals, on the legal minimum scope for the assessment. However, it will still primarily be the responsibility of the developer to seek such advice to ensure that the scope of the EIA is adequately defined. The Environment Agency have recently introduced a set of scoping guides[19] which place considerable emphasis on consensus in the planning of sensitive areas. Nevertheless, effective scoping reduces unnecessary expenditure on researching issues which are of less relevance to decision making and enables limited resources to be allocated most effectively.

Health should always be one of the issues to be included within the scope of an EIA. If the requirement for including health is couched in only general terms, this will lead to an imprecise and insubstantial coverage within the environmental impact statement. Many EIA consultants' reports include only a vague paragraph about health that typically proposes more health education and more health care provision as the solution to all health problems. This was evident in the review of environmental impact statements undertaken for this report (see Appendix 6). If health is to be recognised as one of the key issues, the scoping process must go further and identify the health components in sufficient detail to ensure that adequate statements about health impacts are made.

The scoping process will identify the project boundaries in both time and geographical space. Some of these boundaries are familiar components of EIAs: air and water discharges may drift far downwind or downstream; river diversions have impacts as far as the open sea. Within these boundaries lie all the human communities or community groups whose health may be affected by the project. They include long distance immigrants and future offspring. The ability of current projects to affect future generations is particularly alarming and such considerations gave rise to the common goal of sustainable development. The assessment should focus on the most vulnerable community groups because if they are safeguarded then everyone else must be. However, defining the "most vulnerable group" of people for each health impact may be difficult. In the case of policy assessments, the boundaries may be global in scope. For example, decisions about power station emissions may affect the entire global climate and threaten the resource base on which human life depends.

Health risks change with time and it is convenient to distinguish the construction, early and late operation and decommissioning or rehabilitation stages of the project. Many health risks have a long latent period and need not affect the community on an appreciable scale until ten or twenty years into the future. Cancers, reproductive abnormalities and neurological disorders are examples of health impacts that may have a long delay and multiple causes.[20] Traumatic injuries are examples of health impacts which have little or no delay.

2.1   Identifying health hazards

During the scoping process a detailed list is drawn up of the health hazards that should be investigated. The source of information about these hazards is similar to that for screening, but more detailed and will include experience of similar projects elsewhere, opinions of specialists involved in the scoping process, the concerns of the community and community leaders, other stakeholders, reference documents, maps and national health data.

Identification of health hazards needs to be systematic and comprehensive. For example, some EIAs of reservoir projects have limited health hazard identification to water-related diseases and take no account of the many other potential and important health impacts associated with such projects.

There are currently no comprehensive checklists of the human health hazards that could be consulted during the scoping process. However, there are a number of systematic reviews of the literature that identify known health hazards within each sector.[21,22,23]

The two components of screening and scoping together represent the first of the three objectives to be accomplished by including health in EIA, namely:

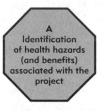

2.2 Categories of health hazard for identification during screening and scoping steps

The health of a community at a particular time is usually assessed by epidemiologists, using portfolios of health indicators. These most commonly measure varying combinations of life expectancy, mortality, morbidity and quality of life and estimate the frequency of various kinds of ill-health in the community. Typical examples are infant mortality rate and the frequency of hospital admissions with particular diseases. When diseases are of specific concern there are often special surveys and these provide limited, but more accurate statistics. Annual summaries are published by the Chief Medical Officer with the title "On the state of the public health". In this report we are supposing that if a survey of health indicators were conducted before and after implementation of an action (whether policy, programme or project), and all other influences could be excluded, then changes in those variables would provide an indication of the impact of that action. The assessment process attempts to predict, for decision-making purposes, the direction of that change. The process also identifies mitigation measures to ensure that, on average, the change should be beneficial, or at least neutral, but not harmful.

Health hazards may arise from a number of different sources, eg biological, chemical, physical and psychological. Unfortunately, there is no comprehensive methodology in the UK for addressing the potential health hazards of a project. As a starting point for discussion and UK methodology development, the potential health hazards arising from a project may be grouped into five main categories. These categories are based on a model developed by Birley,[24] as follows:

- Communicable disease, eg sexually transmitted diseases, infections, and microbiological food contamination.
- Non-communicable disease, eg chronic poisoning, lung disease associated with dust, noise, vibration etc.
- Inappropriate nutrition, eg deprivation, access to food, pesticide or other chemical contamination.
- Injury, eg traffic injury, violence resulting from inner city decay, occupational injury.
- Mental disorder, eg stress, chronic depression and substance abuse.

Each of these working categories is discussed below. These working categories should be taken as a basis for developing comprehensive HIA methodology for the UK. Some of the categories necessarily overlap eg, microbiological contamination of food has been placed in the 'communicable disease' category (in accordance with PHLS classification of salmonella and E-Coli contamination as communicable diseases) rather than under 'inappropriate nutrition'. Other categories may be added, such as the special risks to pregnant women; the developing foetus; and the growth and development of children, which are the subject of a separate study by the British Medical Association. Categories for indirect impacts on health such as those arising from social impacts should also be included in developing HIA methodology. Social impacts may be negative eg, loss of amenity, severance of communities, or positive eg, reduction in unemployment.

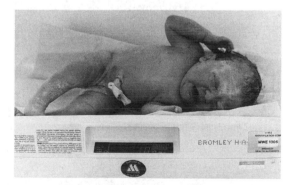

Particular health hazards may affect the growth and development of children

2.2.1 Communicable disease

Respiratory infection, gastro-intestinal infection and malaria remain the most frequent causes of severe morbidity in many developing countries. In the UK, however, many of the communicable diseases found in developing countries are encountered less frequently, if at all. The last 20 years have, for example, witnessed a significant and welcome reduction in the frequency of tuberculosis, despite some new outbreaks of the infection that have been associated both with poverty and with HIV infections, particularly in the United States but also in parts of the UK.[25] The incidence of bacterial infection of surgical wounds has been reduced as a result of modern aseptic techniques, laminar flow operating theatre environments, and the prophylactic use of antibiotics. Even so, some wound contamination from resident skin bacteria or from nasal commensal organisms such as Staphylococci is almost inevitable. Methicillin sensitive Staphylococcus aureus (MSSA) may be isolated from asymptomatic people, but it has the potential to cause infections of skin, wounds, intravenous sites, etc, leading in some cases to the spread of infection with subsequent illness and death.

The development of multiple drug resistant Staphylococcus aureus (MRSA) has caused problems in an increasing number of hospitals.[26] For such infections, the choice of antibiotic agents is limited to a much smaller number of drugs, with problems of cost and toxicity. In addition, the strains of MRSA which are currently being encountered can be spread very easily from person to person. It is therefore particularly important to control the carriage of MRSA within hospitals, to prevent the infections that would otherwise occur in a small proportion of those who acquire the organism. Elderly or debilitated patients, or those in special units such as intensive care or transplants units, are particularly at risk.

Guidelines for the control of MRSA, published in 1990,[27] are due to be updated. They cover the screening of staff in certain circumstances, with possible treatment and exclusion from work, although the MRSA problem is not 'caused' by staff carriers, but rather they have become carriers as a result of working in an environment where MRSA is present. The role of staff screening is still under discussion in the medical literature.[28,29,30,31] It may be better to instill good basic practice, and concentrate on those who might have infections or infected skin conditions which could represent a source of MRSA. At present screening is neither routine nor extensive, but it is sometimes desirable for epidemiological purposes.

The incidence of gastro-intestinal food-borne and water-borne infections is greatly affected by factors such as water engineering, food storage and food handling. Many parasitic, bacterial and viral disease hazards associated with the tropics are now rare in the UK as a result of vigilant health protection agencies or immunisation programmes. They include tapeworm and hydatid parasites, poliomyelitis and the childhood diseases such as measles and rubella.

Food contamination and food scares have received much public attention in recent years. Cases of Salmonella in England and Wales have increased significantly over the last decade and the incidence of E-Coli 0157 is also increasing. Although the rates of E-Coli are variable throughout the UK, Scotland has reported the highest rate of incidence. In 1996, the Public Health Laboratory Service documented ten outbreaks of E-Coli in England and Wales involving 660 confirmed cases. People became infected through the consumption of contaminated foods, particularly inadequately cooked minced beef and dairy produce.[32] The issue of Bovine Spongiform Encephalopathy (BSE) has given rise to great public concern about food safety, and there is mistrust in relation to government action in this area. The BMA recommended the establishment of an independent Ministry of Food to address the conflict of interest inherent in MAFF arising from its role in regulating the food production industry and its responsibilities towards the public in relation to food safety.[33] The proposed establishment of the Food Standards Agency is therefore welcomed.[34] The Agency will have a key role to play in relation to food-borne illnesses and food hygiene. Consumers need to be confident that foodstuffs purchased have been produced to the highest standards and stored correctly prior to consumption. This includes re-education of the public about the basic rules of preservation, food handling and preparation.

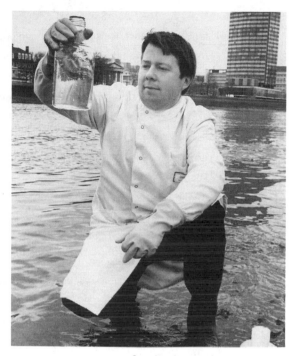

Sampling for waterborne infections

The Food Standards Agency should undertake a thorough review of food safety legislation. Much legislation has been put in place in relation to European Directives and to food scares within the UK. Health impact assessment in relation to food safety would ensure that food legislation and future policy are effective and that there is clear guidance for industry and the consumer, along with sufficient funds for inspection and monitoring.

Sexually transmitted diseases (STDs), including hepatitis B and HIV, are threats to public health in all countries and a particular concern in relation to projects that are major employers of migrant labour, such as the construction of roads. When preparing an HIA for such developments, the risk of STDs should be taken into account so that appropriate health information can be provided to workers.

2.2.2 Non-communicable disease

Cancers, lung disease associated with dust, air pollution, noise, vibration; and chronic poisoning are hazards associated with projects such as agro-chemicals, road construction, quarrying and mining. Exposure may occur at places of both work and residence through unregulated emissions to the air, soil or water and through inappropriate use of machinery. For example, asbestosis and mesothelioma are associated with asbestos exposure and afflict both those who manufacture products containing the mineral and those who use the products. In contrast to communicable diseases, the source of hazardous material may be localised.

There has been an increase of about 50% in the prevalence of childhood asthma over the last 30 years and data from the Department of Health reveal that hospital admissions for the condition have increased from 4,000 in 1980 to 10,000 in 1990.[35] It has been suggested that these trends are related to air pollution, with the proposal that air pollution could both initiate asthma in previously healthy individuals or aggravate or provoke symptoms in those already asthmatic.

The Department of Health Committee on the Medical Effects of Air Pollutants (COMEAP) reviewed the available evidence to determine whether asthma and outdoor air pollution are in fact linked.[36] The Committee concluded that the available evidence did not support a causative role for outdoor air pollution. However, in relation to worsening or provocation of symptoms it was concluded that only a small proportion of patients may experience a clinically significant effect. There may also be a link between perceived air

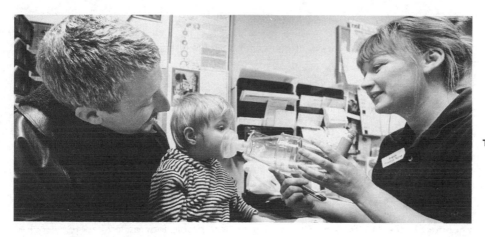

Traffic volumes may be linked to childhood respiratory symptoms including asthma

quality and psychosomatic symptoms which have been associated with recurrent colds and chronic bronchitis, including among school children.[37]

A number of studies have found correlations between neighbourhood traffic volumes and child respiratory symptoms, including hospital admissions for asthma.[38,39] However, despite the evidence for the health risks associated with air pollution, Government departments have taken a short-term view (ten years) of road traffic air pollution, coinciding with the predicted decline in emissions up to 2005 associated with catalytic converters. The projected increase in traffic after 2005 will, however, negate the benefits won by catalytic converters.

A further study was carried out by the Department of Health Committee on the Medical Effects of Air Pollutants (COMEAP) to investigate air pollution exposure-response relationships.[40] The committee concluded that for air pollution there is no safe threshold of effect, and that even low levels of exposure may adversely affect those in high risk groups, eg people suffering from respiratory disease such as asthma. The report emphasised the importance of estimating the costs of air pollution on health in the UK.

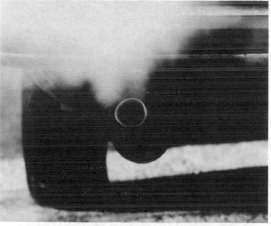

Vehicle exhaust contains a number of pollutants and can aggravate respiratory diseases

2.2.3   Inappropriate nutrition

This is a particular sub-category of non-communicable disease that is perceived to be an important consequence of new policies and so may conveniently be identified separately. Many policies are likely to have an impact on the food security and nutritional status of certain vulnerable communities through a variety of indirect and unplanned mechanisms. These include food production, food availability, workload, and feeding practices. In the developing world, changes in land use may deprive subsistence peoples of wild foods, cash economies may alter the food entitlements within households and increased burdens on carers may reduce the time available for cooking.

While the consequences of over-eating and poor balance of diet are more important in the UK than are those of acute or chronic lack of food more typical of developing countries, the latter have become more evident in recent times.[41] The linkage between economic well-being and health is clear: communities with adequate incomes can afford to eat balanced diets and to live more healthy lifestyles. Those with incomes which are less adequate are vulnerable to both communicable and non-communicable diseases.

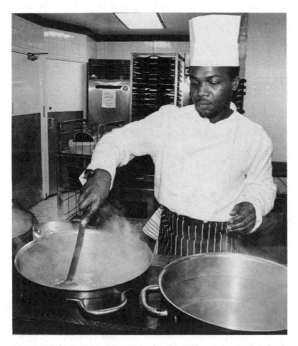

The use of land for roads, private housing, out of town constructions (eg supermarkets, industrial estates etc) has been accompanied by a decline in land available for allotments and small holdings which have traditionally been a source of fresh food. Out of town supermarkets, with their associated closure of local shops and markets, have taken the place of such traditional food sources. Increasing motorisation has also encouraged the siting of supermarkets on the outskirts of towns, which are often served by few or no public transport routes. Those who have no access to a car must shop at the generally more expensive local shops which have reduced their range of stock in order to compete. This may lead to diminished access to

Many policies have an impact on food security and nutritional status, particularly of vulnerable communities

fresh, nutritious, basic foods for the elderly and urban poor. If people are unable to get easy access to the right food, they may eat convenience food, leading to chronic deficiency in essential nutrients. Health impact assessment at the appropriate planning stage could help to direct retail developments to deprived urban areas, outlying housing estates and remote settlements. The problems of inappropriate nutrition should be addressed within the Green Paper *Our Healthier Nation*[42] and are included in the remit of the proposed Food Standards Agency.[43] It is important that good eating habits are established in childhood, since prevention of illnesses such as coronary heart disease and cancers[44] need to be addressed at an early age. The introduction of nutritional standards for school meals would correct inappropriate nutrition caused by past policies and have a major role to play in the health of children and subsequent generations.

2.2.4 Injury

Human injury is caused by the rapid interchange of mechanical, thermal, radiant, chemical or electrical energy with the human body. While road deaths and serious casualties are declining in the UK (3,598 people were killed and 44,473 seriously injured in 1996),[45] speed has been recognised for some years to be a key determinant of road injuries and severity.[46,47] Communal violence is a frequent problem of displacement, overcrowding and inner city decay. In developing countries the urban centres are surrounded by shanty towns that are subject to fire, flood and landslides. Occupational safety is a recurrent theme of all industrial processes; safety standards are difficult to enforce and labour is not always mindful of the hazards. Mining, quarrying and deep sea diving are frequently hazardous. Explosions are a severe but infrequent hazard of modern industry because of increased awareness of hazards and the provision of adequate safety measures.

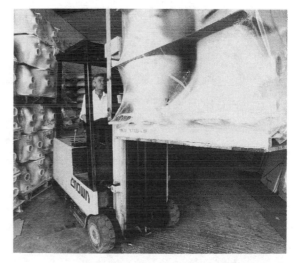

Occupational injury is an important category of health hazard

2.2.5   Mental disorder

There is little hard information available about the association of mental disorder and psycho-social well-being with development projects and policies. Stress, chronic depression and substance abuse are apparent consequences of excessive noise and vibration,[48,49] urbanisation and unemployment resulting from projects and policies. Shift workers may experience mental disorder associated with loss of biological rhythm,[50] affecting their ability to avoid injury to themselves and others when working with complex or fast moving machinery. Other problems associated with stress include suicide, violent behaviour and eating disorders.[51] The loss of well-being associated with the pace of modern life may not cause measurable morbidity, but is a concern to many people. Mental health is a key area of *Our Healthier Nation*.[52] The 1995 *Health Survey for England* showed that 20% of women and 14% of men may have had a mental illness;[53] and mental disorders accounted for 15% and 26% of days of certified incapacity in the early 1990s in men and women respectively. The methods and approaches of social impact assessment may facilitate investigations of psycho-social well-being, and these should be integrated with health assessment.

During the last 20 years there has been a renewed recognition of the health impact of housing conditions and policies. Mental health aspects include the stress caused by overcrowding; by noise; and by structural problems such as dampness. Mental health related problems associated with public sector flat dwelling, in addition to those already mentioned, include vandalism, poorly maintained lifts, badly designed and lit stairwells and hallways, and inappropriate allocation of families with young children to flats.[54] Mental illness and psychoneurotic problems are more common among young mothers who live in flats than those who live elsewhere.

The causes of poor mental health are complex; however, the Government has identified the following environmental factors, and proposes to improve mental health by: continuing to invest in housing and reduce homelessness; encouraging employers to address workplace stress; reducing isolation through transport policy, and promoting healthy schools.[55]

2.3   Considering alternatives

As with other components of the impact assessment, it is crucial that planning for the assessment takes place at an early stage in the project cycle so that preliminary plans can be modified if necessary, to safeguard human health. For example, project siting can determine the exposure of communities to air or water-borne discharges and also increased traffic. Assessments that take place too late in the planning cycle may lose the opportunity to consider alternatives. It is common for a project to treat effluent to an agreed standard and then make unrealistic assumptions about what happens to the effluent after it leaves their site and ceases to be their responsibility. Extreme cases are seen in developing countries where wastewater containing pathogens and heavy metals may be used for irrigation.[56] About 50% of the water-borne sewage produced in India is used for irrigation of crops.[57] Effective EIA should help to ensure that good decisions are made about the siting and design of new developments on environmental and health grounds. It will fail to achieve this unless consideration of alternatives is given due emphasis early in the EIA process. In the UK, alternative sites and designs are rarely assessed in detail, making it very difficult to optimise planning choices. A thorough discussion of alternatives should ensure that the developer has considered other possible approaches to the project, as well as available means of minimising negative environmental and health impacts. It enables EIAs to provide a framework for the competent authority's decision, rather than justification for one particular action. Finally, if unforeseen difficulties arise during construction or operation of a project, a re-examination of the alternatives may help to identify possible

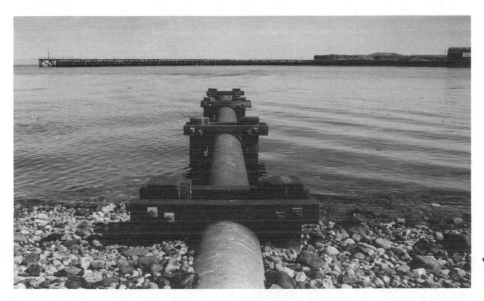

Project siting should take account of exposure of communities to water-borne discharges

solutions. The consideration of alternatives was not a mandatory requirement of the original European EIA Directive[58] and as a consequence is discretionary under the present UK regulations. However, the new Directive[59] now makes it compulsory for the developers to include "at least an outline of the main alternatives studied by the developer and an indication of the main reasons for this choice, taking into account the environmental effects." This revision must be incorporated into the UK regulations by March 1999.

3.   Terms of reference

Once the health hazards associated with the project have been identified by the screening and scoping components of the EIA process, the next step is the production of the Terms of Reference (TOR) for the consultant who will carry out the assessment. The Terms of Reference are likely to stipulate the required contents of the environmental impact statement (EIS) which will be submitted with the planning application. As noted earlier, scoping benefits from full and early discussion between the developer, the relevant competent authority, other relevant agencies and authorities, affected parties and interest groups. This enables the extent of available information to be ascertained and knowledge gaps identified and filled.

A crucial issue that arises out of all examinations of environmental impact statements (EISs) for health components is that consultants will only report what is required by their Terms of Reference. If only vague questions are asked about health, the outputs obtained will be unclear and general.

3.1   Including health in the terms of reference

The terms of reference need to be specific about how the consultant should assess the health risks associated with the health hazards already identified at the scoping stage, as well as requiring the consultant to include any other hazards encountered during the study. The elements of health impact assessment that should be addressed by the consultants include:

- Listing potential health hazards through a scoping process, sub-divided into categories of communicable disease, non-communicable disease, inappropriate nutrition, injury and mental disorders;

- Identifying potentially vulnerable communities and describing why they are vulnerable;
- Identifying the environmental factors responsible for exposure of vulnerable communities to hazards;
- Describing the capacities and capabilities of the many agencies responsible for protecting health in relation to the project and identifying their limitations;
- Reaching a conclusion based on the above regarding the change in health risk reasonably attributable to the project ranked at least as a trend of increasing/decreasing or no change;
- Recommending health safeguards and mitigation measures in sufficient detail to be given serious consideration, including outline costs.

Guidelines and statutory requirements are needed to ensure that these components are included within EISs. The review of EISs commissioned by the BMA for this report proposed 'lack of explicit legislation' as one possible explanation for the inadequate coverage of health hazards (see Appendix 6).

3.2   Consultation

Lack of early consultation and discussion is a major limitation to effective EIA, and consultation should take place as early as possible and continue throughout the EIA process to ensure that important information is not missed out and all relevant interests and aspects are explored. The DETR recommends that developers should consult with the competent authority and statutory consultees before preparing the EIS, but in practice this happens in only about half of all cases. The benefits of early consultation were highlighted by an assessment of flood defence proposals for Newtownards in Northern Ireland for which extensive consultation was undertaken at the scoping stage. At the initial consultation stage a scoping document was sent to some 29 organisations, with special presentations made to key groups. A scoping report was then prepared and a more detailed secondary consultation stage was undertaken which involved the establishment of a small working group. The group represented major interests and members were chosen for their specialism and perceived ability to 'represent' areas of concern. Three meetings were held during which the issues and alternative options were considered. It proved to be a valuable tool for public participation. The provision of a clear remit for the working group, with agreed terms of reference and time-tabled meetings was found to be effective. Ideally the consultations and working group proceedings should be published to provide reassurance that the issues of concern to the public have been raised and addressed.[60]

Early consultation therefore plays an important part in determining the final terms of reference of an EIA. A further example comes from Australia, where the proponent of the proposed third runway at Sydney (Kingsford Smith) Airport sought the guidance of both federal and the New South Wales government. Draft terms of reference were made available for public comment as part of the early consultation process. After only one month more than 250 submissions were received from the public and considered before finalising the terms of reference for the consultants carrying out the EIA.

It is the responsibility of the development proponent to ensure that due consultation has been made with the relevant statutory consultees in compiling the EIS for a planning proposal. The Environment Agency has replaced Her Majesty's Inspectorate of Pollution (HMIP) as statutory consultee in circumstances where a proposal involves "works specified in Schedule 1 to the Health and Safety (Emissions to the Atmosphere) Regulations 1983".[61] In addition, planning authorities are expected to consult with the Health and Safety Executive in circumstances where a proposed development involves "the manufacture, processing, keeping or use of a hazardous substance in such circumstances that there will at any one time be, or is likely to be, a notifiable quantity of such substance in, on, over or under any land."[62] However, there is no statutory consultee for remaining health-related issues, increasing the risk of their omission from the EIA process.

The decision-making authority will also undertake consultation to gauge the adequacy of information provided in an EIS. The statutory consultees, the public or the planning authority may wish to see modifications to the project design, or additional measures to mitigate any adverse effects. The planning authorities have a certain amount of power to enforce such measures through planning conditions and therefore have a very important part to play in promoting 'best practice' in EIA and in ensuring that health impacts are taken into account. It is important to note that their ability to evaluate any health impacts which are identified may be hampered by a lack of relevant expertise. Effective consultation with environmental health specialists in local authorities and with Directors of Public Health at an early stage and throughout the EIA process is therefore important.

The new EIA Directive[63] places greater emphasis on consultation throughout the EIA process. In particular, "Member States shall ensure that any request for development and any information gathered [as part of the EIA] are made available to the public within a reasonable time in order to give the public concerned the opportunity to express an opinion before the development consent is granted". Furthermore, "when a decision to grant or refuse development consent has been taken, the competent authority or authorities shall inform the public ... and make available to the public the following information: the content of the decision and any conditions attached thereto; the main reasons and considerations on which the decision is based; a description, where necessary, of the main measures to avoid, reduce and, if possible, offset any major adverse effects".

A further addition reflects the requirements of the Espoo Convention on Transboundary EIA, that consultation must also be undertaken with the public and environmental authorities in neighbouring Member States if they are likely to be affected by the project (known as transboundary effects). In implementing the new EIA Directive, the UK Government supports the aims to make the process more open to the public but is concerned that this scrutiny is not cost-effective for minor development projects which have no significant effects within the meaning of the Directive. 'Exclusive' thresholds are therefore proposed, below which projects would not be required to undergo such public scrutiny (see Figure 3).[64]

4. Preparing the EIS

Once the TORs have been completed and consulted, the next stage is to prepare the EIS. The main task of the consultant in producing the EIS is:

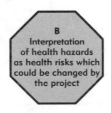

**Figure 4: The main components of the
assessment of change in health risk**

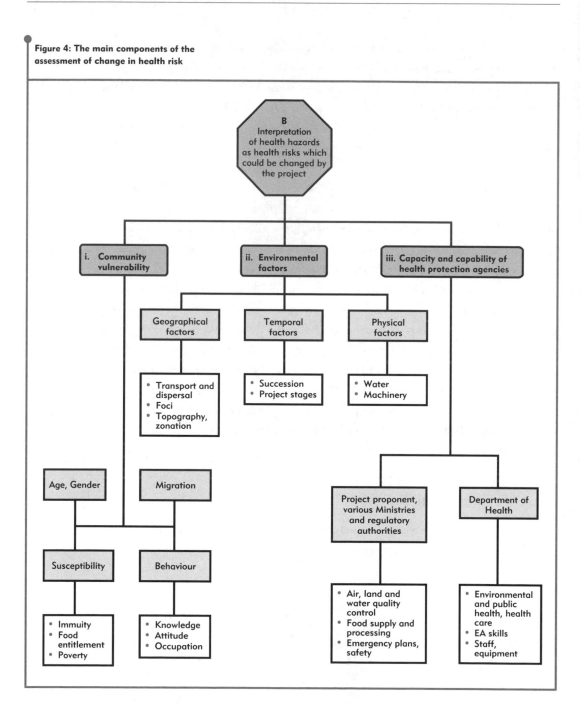

This is the second objective to be accomplished by including health in the EIA process. There is no universally accepted methodology for this. Experience suggests that the problem can be divided into three essential components and that these should receive explicit attention in the TOR (see Figure 4). These components for the assessment of health risks are:

i. **Community vulnerability** — identifying the communities affected by the project and determining how they are vulnerable (ie health effects);

ii. **Environmental factors** — identifying the environmental factors that expose the vulnerable communities to the health hazards;

iii. **Health protection agencies** — analysing the capacity and capability of health protection agencies to safeguard the communities.

Each of these main components is discussed below and each can be sub-divided into further levels of detail.

4.1   Community vulnerability

In contrast to an EIA which focuses on the environment, a health assessment puts the human community first and complements other approaches such as social impact assessment. The community is composed of a number of groups who differ in their vulnerability to health hazards; the range of factors affecting vulnerability may include age and sex of the subject, the amount of exercise taken, whether a woman is pregnant, her susceptibility and behaviour. Determining the risk to a foetus is particularly problematic as hazards which normally pose little or no threat to the general population may cause harm to the foetus. For example, exposure of pregnant women to substances such as lead and mercury has been linked with birth defects.[65] The communities first need to be identified and then their vulnerabilities described. The communities themselves are important sources of information about their existing health problems and health concerns. A person may be more susceptible because of their immune or nutritional status. These, in turn, are affected by pre-existing diseases, state of health, pregnancy and other factors. Inappropriate behaviour is partly the result of poor knowledge, attitude or belief and can be identified by simple community surveys. Community survey methods need to be extended to combine vulnerability to health hazards together with perception of and attitudes to risk in different

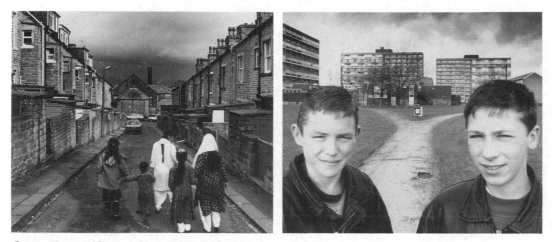

Communities may differ in their vulnerability to health hazards

communities. Important forms of behaviour include health care seeking, hazard avoidance and dietary habits. Poverty and occupation are contributing factors.

Voluntary, community and tenants' groups should be consulted appropriately - and will frequently act as powerful advocates for their community's health and social interests. Within the National Health Service, Community Health Councils (Local Health Councils in Scotland) may serve a similar function. The appropriate community group to address may change as the programme, policy or project develops. During the construction stage, the community may consist largely of single adult males. During the operational stage it may include formally employed workers of both sexes and members of a service sector, eg cleaners.

Examples of community vulnerability:
- Compulsory use of car safety belts has reduced the frequency of severe traffic injuries, illustrating how behaviour affects vulnerability.
- Immunisation policies reduce the frequency of certain communicable diseases, illustrating how susceptibility affects vulnerability.
- Dose-response relationships to hazardous substances vary with age and gender so that small children may be more vulnerable to a given dose of a toxin than adults, eg exposure to lead.[66]
- As inequalities in income and living standards have increased in the UK so have mortality differentials, illustrating that poverty contributes to vulnerability.[67]

4.2   Environmental factors

The environment is an important determinant of exposure of vulnerable people to health hazards. It includes the natural and the man-made environment. In rural settings, for example, a farming project can promote development of a succession of plant and animal communities, including agricultural pests and weeds. In the urban areas, development may affect the built environment such as roads and housing. Environmental factors may lead to problems of drainage and solid waste disposal. Chemical pollutants are transported through various media, eg air, water and soil, and geological factors affect the transport of pollutants. Natural topography determines the direction of dispersal. Land use patterns affect the exposure of people, for example, zones may be established for different uses such as residential, agricultural and industrial which can help to separate people from pollutants. In the working environment, injury is caused by fast moving machinery and poisoning by exposure to hazardous substances. Noise is a common problem of both the work and domestic environments.

Example of environmental factors:
Chemicals may contaminate groundwater as a result of dumping, accidental spillage or leaching from landfill sites. The groundwater may then be used as a source of drinking water.[68,69]

The environmental factors responsible for hazard exposure can be identified and categorised as:

- focal or dispersed,
- frequent or infrequent,
- near or distant.

Risk or industrial hazard assessment is a component of health assessment that focuses almost exclusively on the environmental factors. It often involves an engineering analysis of the concentration of an unintended release of energy or chemical at various distances from a point source and the probability of that release occurring. Many environmental concerns have been driven by the perceived risk to human health of hazardous chemicals. There are about 70,000 chemicals in daily use[70] and the number is

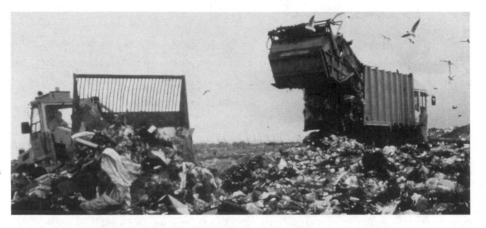

Chemicals may contaminate groundwater as a result of leaching from landfill sites

increasing by about 1,000 per year.[71] Substances may be taken up through respiration, ingestion or absorption (see Figure 5). Dose-response evaluation involves the characterisation of the relationship between the dose of a chemical administered or received and the incidence or severity of an adverse health effect in the exposed individual or population. People are exposed to toxic chemicals through a variety of mechanisms, including the following:

- Direct exposure to high concentrations of a toxic chemical occurs through intentional and unintentional releases.

- Secondary poisoning occurs when a chemical accumulates as it passes through the ecosystem, even though it may have been released at concentrations that were considered harmless. Chemicals to which people would not normally be exposed may also be transformed by biological or chemical processes in the environment into forms which can then become 'bioavailable', that is to say they can be absorbed.

- Indirect effects occur when the toxic chemical pollutes resources, such as food or water supplies.

- Multiple exposure effects occur when a person is exposed to many different chemicals, each of which may have been released at a safe concentration. The consequence of exposure to a mixture of chemicals may be by summation of the action of each component, or sometimes the components may interact, causing a different and usually enhanced effect.

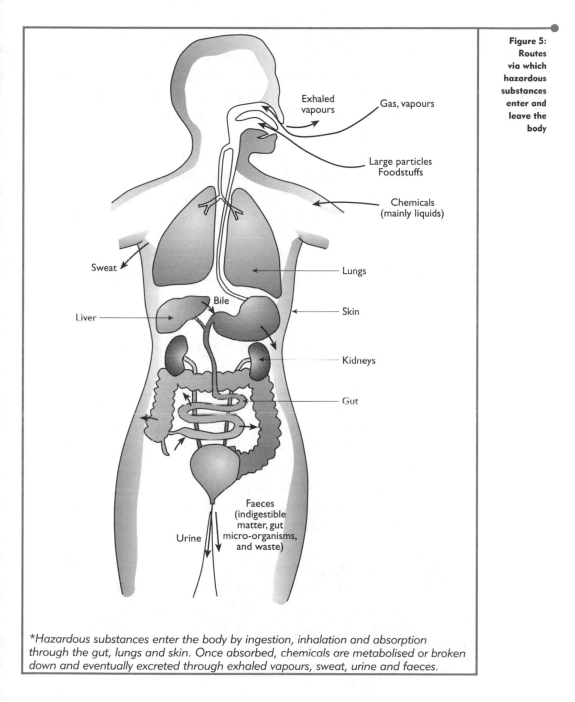

Figure 5: Routes via which hazardous substances enter and leave the body

Hazardous substances enter the body by ingestion, inhalation and absorption through the gut, lungs and skin. Once absorbed, chemicals are metabolised or broken down and eventually excreted through exhaled vapours, sweat, urine and faeces.

If someone were to encounter a mixture of simple irritants, such as, for example, formaldehyde and acid vapours, the inflammation caused in the skin, eyes or upper respiratory tract would usually be additive. However, the inhalation of a combination of sulphur dioxide and airborne particles, as in smog, will lead to increased irritation, probably because the acid gas is adsorbed onto the particles so that a larger amount is carried further down the airways. As little is known about the health effects of mixed exposure cases, the best general approach is always to consider the possibility of interactions when evaluating the potential harmfulness of a mixed exposure by taking account of the toxic load and properties of the individual components and their interactions.

4.3   Capacity and capability of health protection agencies

Protection of human health is the responsibility of many agencies including the Department of Health, Department of the Environment, Transport and the Regions, Department of Trade and Industry, the Health and Safety Executive, planning authorities and the many companies, inspectorates and monitoring agencies associated with the water industry. The role of some of these agencies was discussed in Chapter 2. Health activities are also undertaken by a range of non-governmental organisations and the private sector is also an important source of health care. Another important source of health protection is the project proponent itself. The environment and health impact assessment should determine whether these agencies have the capacity and capability to prevent exposure of the vulnerable community to the identified health hazards or to care for them after they are exposed. Capacity refers to resources in terms of staff, equipment, communications, and transport. Capability refers to the skills of the staff to use their resources.

Example of capacity and capability of health protection agencies:

The BMA publication, *Hazardous Waste and Human Health*[72] provided examples of the under-staffing in waste disposal and monitoring authorities which limits their capacity to prevent unsafe hazardous waste disposal practices even though there are well-developed laws and regulations for this purpose.

In its report on the environmental and occupational risks of health care,[73] the BMA expressed concern that less than 15% of all companies in the UK have access to occupational health services. It was also noted that the Government planned substantial reduction in expenditure by the Health and Safety Executive amounting to more than £10M per year. This was set against the estimated cost of accidents which is £16 billion per year.

If a project creates new or unusual health risks, the staff of health protection agencies will need additional training on how best to respond. The assessment should determine whether a multi-sectoral approach is taken towards planning. For example, are there any formal or informal linkages between the various agencies and the project proponent?

4.4   Drawing conclusions regarding change in health risk

The three components of the heath risk assessment described above (sections 4.1-4.3) provide the basis for the conclusion of the EIS regarding the change in a health risk that can reasonably be attributed to the project.

Ideally, the conclusion would be both qualitative and quantitative. In practice, this depends on the quality of the numerical data and the availability of a model that combines the components. In the absence of such data and models, a simpler ranking of trend may be all that is practicable. This consists of a statement, for each health hazard, vulnerable community and project stage, that a change in health risk is attributable to the project. The conclusion should also state whether the change is an increase or decrease in the health risk. In order to improve communication with the many stakeholders, the conclusion could be presented in several stages of increasing detail:

- summary table, such as Table 3. The number of rows can be expanded to include all the health hazards.
- summary justifications of the statements included in the table.
- more detailed presentations of the data and the assumptions on which the justifications are based.

**Table 3: Model summary
health assessment table**

Health hazard	Community group	Vulnerability of community group	Environmental factors determining exposure to the hazard	Capacity and capability of health protection agencies	Change in health risk attributable to the project
Communicable diseases					
Non-communicable diseases					
Injury					
Inappropriate nutrition					
Mental disorder					

4.4.1   Assessment of health risks

Assessment and evaluation of hazards and risks depend on the gathering of data, and the processing of them by various means. The way data (and information derived from it) are processed differs between different groups of stakeholders.

Scientists tend to believe they arrive at an assessment of risks by interpreting data in the light of their understanding of the processes and mechanisms that determine how the world works. Industry, and regulatory bodies, need to operate as efficiently as possible, and make decisions on the basis of risk assessment systems which use relatively small amounts of data to calculate relative risk. These groups cope with uncertainty by applying quite large safety factors in the risk assessment process. Losses in efficiency are compensated by continued effectiveness in keeping risks low. The general public make judgements about risks based on their perception of a situation. The view they form of a risk or hazard is conditioned by social and political factors. One of the most important of these is the trust they have in the experts providing interpretations of the data from which risks need to be assessed; another important factor is probably the openness of the risk assessment and evaluation process. Communicating risks is therefore complex, particularly as terminology is often inconsistent. A system of standardising the terminology has been proposed by the Chief Medical Officer[74] which, if adopted, could prove of great assistance to public and professionals alike.

The conclusion regarding health risk is reached from a synthesis of the information gathered during the analysis of the essential components. The summary health assessment table will assist in that synthesis and in the communication of the results. There will be many uncertainties and assumptions will have to be made, and it is important that uncertainties and ignorance are explicitly acknowledged. Assumptions are only appropriate if they are stated explicitly so that those responsible for review/appraisal of the EIS are able to make a judgement about their value, in the light of the information from which the assumptions are derived.

All available methods of assessment rely on a degree of expert judgement. This is reasonable provided that values and assumptions are clearly stated so that the reader is free to agree or disagree. All methods also rely on comparisons with previous completed projects of a similar type in a similar region. Information about such projects is usually incomplete and no two projects are exactly alike and so the differences between projects should be acknowledged as well as the similarities.[75]

Health impact assessment should aim to be holistic and harvest the opinion of as many relevant experts as possible. Lack of data and uncertainty must be accepted as inevitable components of the process. Each new assessment throws up questions that are amenable to research studies; but the outcome of such research is only usually available in time to contribute to future assessments.

The conclusions of the health impact assessment will prompt debate and decisions for health risk mitigation. They will be used by proponents and opponents of the project or policy for their own political ends and many may feel that the only acceptable level of risk is 'no risk'. Much work remains to educate the public and politicians in risk interpretation.[76]

4.4.2 Toxicology and public health

Estimates of the impact of environmental agents on health require information on exposure and on the quantitative relationship between exposure and effects on health. Precise estimates of exposure are rarely possible, however, owing to the scarcity of monitoring data. The estimates of exposure are, therefore, based on limited information and, whenever feasible, supplemented by extrapolations based on some reasonable assumptions; the resulting uncertainties may be considerable.

Preparation of an EIA may draw upon toxicological data. Toxicology can be defined as the study of poisons, with special reference to their preparation, identification, physiological action and antidotes.[77] Environmental toxicology enjoys the same principles as toxicology and is concerned with agents which contaminate or are purposely added to food, air, water, soil and the working place.[78] However, knowledge of the effects on human health of various exposures, based on toxicological studies, is far from complete. This leads to further uncertainties.[79]

When a toxicologist investigates the potential impact of a substance on the environment, the hazard must first be detected before an assessment of the risk is made. The sequence of steps in assessing the risk is as follows:

- Identify the hazard;
- Identify the population at risk;
- Characterise the hazard by investigating its nature, the route of exposure (ie inhalation, ingestion or skin contact) and the dose (time) response relation;
- Determine or predict that population's exposure;
- Predict outcome.[80]

In general, the severity of the impact on health is assumed to depend on the extent of the exposure and the corresponding dose of the environmental agent, but the precise dose-relationship is often not known. For some environmental agents, doses below a certain threshold level can be accommodated and are not harmful. Others, such as allergens, ionizing radiation and chemical genotoxic carcinogens, are believed to have no threshold dose and to pose a risk at all levels of exposure. A hazard is defined in this context as the potential of a physical or chemical agent to do harm and a risk is the probability that harm will be done under a given set of circumstances. For some chemicals there are known dose-response functions that describe the proportion of a population that would suffer particular effects for a given exposure. In the case of multiple exposure the effects may be additive or synergistic and new dose-response functions may be required for each combination of chemicals. The cumulative effects of low level exposure may be particularly difficult to determine. In addition, human response to environmental factors is not homogeneous in the population, since some people are more susceptible than others. The source of increased susceptibility may be genetic predisposition, but coexisting environmental or lifestyle factors are also known to influence the response.[81] The dose-response model may also be useful for assessing aspects of inappropriate nutrition, injury and mental disorder, but it is usually not suitable for communicable diseases.

The manner in which the identified risks are managed may differ according to what remedial action is considered feasible, generally acceptable and economic.[82] The risk should be assessed in terms of how many individuals will be affected (both absolute numbers or incidence) and what the harmful effects on them could be. At this stage the toxicologist may consider that his professional task has been completed, and he can leave others to decide on the acceptability and management of the risk which has been identified. This means balancing the personal, public and financial benefits of a new substance or procedure against individual, community, societal and environmental costs. These wider social and economic issues are discussed further in Chapter 5.

4.4.3 The value of exposure standards

For some chemicals, exposure standards have been established and the impact assessment should be concerned with the frequency with which they will be exceeded by particular communities. However, at present, the number of formally adopted standards, eg for chemical exposure, is limited, and despite their existence new and unexpected problems relating to exposure continue to be identified. Adherence to standards mainly helps to protect the public against known health hazards for which data are available. Such data may be derived from laboratory tests which aim to evaluate the risk of exposure to a particular chemical hazard. They are usually carried out by exposing test animals (usually rodents) to a chemical and then monitoring for signs of harm. To limit the expense, the numbers of animals and the time needed, the amounts administered are usually hundreds or thousands of times greater than those a human might normally encounter.

Once the animal data are available, the interpretation of those data involves many assumptions. If a substance is harmful to animals, is it necessarily harmful to humans? If a substance induces no conspicuous adverse effects in the animals, has it been shown to be safe for humans? How can a large dose for a small animal be translated into a small dose for a human? A standard method for evaluating acute chemical toxicity is to report an LD50 value, which is the amount of a substance per kilogram of body weight that is lethal to 50% of the test animals. However, it is extremely difficult, and some would argue impossible, to determine from such data what will be the effects of long-term human exposure to small amounts of the chemical.[83] Furthermore, standards derived from such data often relate to exposure to single chemicals rather than to a mixture of different chemicals which may enhance the effects of each other. The usefulness of standards for chemical exposure is also limited by the fact that they may be set without reference to the way in which the chemical exposure occurs, such as physical contact, inhalation, ingestion.

In contrast, there is no 'standard' person. People have different lifestyles, leading to different exposures, and different susceptibilities to particular hazards. Where they exist, standards are a useful guide as to what might, on average, be expected. Some factors affecting health have no standards attached to them. Standards by themselves are, therefore, not sufficient to assess health impacts.

The United Kingdom National Air Quality Strategy,[84] for example, lists eight pollutants, identified by the Expert Panel on Air Quality Standards (EPAQS), with recommended target maximum levels for each. The report refers to the likely adverse health effects of exposure to pollutants, where these are known. However, where no recommended target level has yet been set by the panel, the air quality standard is that derived from the WHO recommendation and adverse health effects may be less clear (see Appendix 3). The Air Quality Regulations 1997[85] which came into force on 23 December 1997, set the *National Air Quality Strategy* objectives in statutory form and initiated the system of local air quality management under Part IV of the Environment Act 1995. The Government plans to review the *National Air Quality Strategy* in 1998. The review will draw on the findings of the Committee on the Medical Effects of Air Pollutants report on the *Quantification of the Effects of Air Pollution on Health in the United Kingdom*[86] which aimed to define the health effect of air pollution in terms of change in the health of individuals and for the overall population. The Committee concluded that the actual overall effects of air pollution on health in the UK may be higher than their estimates, due to lack of data, particularly for low level effects which may increase levels of overall morbidity. Further work is planned to cost the health impacts of pollution; however, the 1998 report is an important step towards estimating the costs of air pollution in terms of mortality and admissions to hospital. Estimates of health costs, as they develop, may provide data to inform health impact assessments.

4.4.4   Quantifying health risks

Many decision-makers with an engineering or economics background prefer potential impacts to be assigned numerical estimates and economic values, when feasible. There is much debate about the value of quantified methods for assessing health and other impacts. Such methods exist for specific hazards, usually of a physical nature and amenable to engineering analysis. There are methods for determining the response of animals to doses of toxic substances and these can be extrapolated, with increasing uncertainty, to human communities. Retrospective or prospective epidemiological studies can help to assess the relative risk associated with various environmental factors. For example, a review of selected epidemiological studies of acute effects of particulate air pollution showed evidence for increased mortality by approximately 1% per $10\mu g/m^3$ increase in PM_{10} from one day to the next. Morbidity, as measured by respiratory-related hospital admissions and emergency department visits, increased by approximately 0.8% and 1% per $10\mu g/m^3$ PM_{10} respectively.[87] The Committee on the Medical Effects of Air Pollutants[88] attempted to quantify the effects of air pollution on the health of the population of the UK in terms of specific health impacts, such as admission to hospital and advancement of death. The Committee estimated that the deaths of between 12,000 and 24,000 vulnerable people may be brought forward, and between 14,000 and 24,000 hospital admissions and readmissions may be associated with short term air pollution each year.[89] In conclusion,[90] the committee were not able to fully quantify all the effects on mortality; many deaths were associated with days of higher air pollution in the elderly and the sick, and it was likely that air pollutants could hasten the death of such people by a few days or weeks. Long-term exposure to air pollutants at current levels also damages health; however, at present there are insufficient UK data to quantify the effects. The long-term effects of air pollution should be reassessed as data become available. Such data may arise from follow-up monitoring of projects, policies and plans, and from health impact assessments.

There are also dynamic models of some communicable disease systems. These models provide general insights, but cannot predict the outcomes of a specific development project. Many of the linkages between cause and effect are complex and not yet susceptible to detailed numerical analysis.

The opponents of quantified methods point out that decisions are made at many stages in the project cycle and take account of many factors other than purely technical measures of impact.[91] Neither the public nor the politician are attracted to quantification, and risk perception and interpretation is a largely subjective process. Prioritising risks is a political rather than advisory matter which depends on the opinion of stakeholders. Risk aversion varies between stakeholders. For example, there is evidence that people are prepared to accept higher levels of individual voluntary risk than community involuntary risk. Quantification is an important but distant goal, while health safeguards and mitigation measures are required immediately. A very simple ranking of the trend in health risk associated with each health hazard attributable to the project may be all that can be accomplished. Such a ranking might be: no apparent change, increased risk, decreased risk etc. In many cases the ranking will be sufficient for decisions to be made on the basis of the precautionary principle (see 4.4.5 below). Such decisions should include the addition of health risk management measures into the project design, construction, operation and maintenance.

4.4.5   Precautionary principle

In the case of many low level pollutants, it is very difficult or even impossible to establish whether a significant risk exists when a community is exposed to them.[92] Knowledge may be sufficient for taking action, but insufficient to satisfy scientific enquiry.[93] Levels of uncertainty are compounded in conditions of cumulative exposure of many chemicals from many sources. Similar problems exist with new or emergent communicable diseases, such as new variant Creutzfeld-Jakob Disease where the risk of exposure cannot be determined. Under these conditions it is sensible to err on the side of caution (ie adopt a specific interpretation of the precautionary approach). O'Riordan[94] noted that the notion of a 'precautionary principle' can be interpreted in a variety of different ways. The UK government have interpreted it to mean that "where there are significant risks of damage to the environment, the government will be prepared to take precautionary action to limit the use of potentially dangerous materials or the spread of potentially dangerous pollutants, even where scientific knowledge is not conclusive, if the likely balance of costs and benefits justifies it".[95] Use of the precautionary principle helps ensure that decisions made today are not a source of regret tomorrow.

4.4.6 Significance of health risks

The decision to mitigate a health risk or to refuse a project will depend on people's perception of the significance of the potential impacts. Significance can be partly determined by frequency and severity. For example, a health risk which would have a high frequency and would kill people is clearly unacceptable. Similarly, a health risk that has low frequency and causes minor inconvenience is probably acceptable. Health risks with a middle range of severity and frequency may or may not be judged significant.

An important distinction is made between risk estimation and risk evaluation.[96] Health impact assessment is a risk estimation process, however qualitative. Risk evaluation is the social and political process of judging the significance of the risk. One recent report[97] suggested the following general principles for judging a risk to be significant:

- Effects that are irreversible or incurable;
- Involuntary risks (ie, those which are beyond the control of the individual);
- Long-term effects, especially on future generations;
- Substantial impoverishment of the community;
- Substantial reductions in amenity and other quality of life indicators.

Human values, different for each of us, influence our perceptions in such complex ways that it is unlikely that all of us will agree on a single level of acceptable risk.[98,99] Risks have a qualitative as well as a quantitative aspect: some ways of dying are more dreaded than others. Risks and benefits have to be judged together and, of course, problems occur when one community receives the benefits while another community is asked to accept the risks. One method of determining the acceptability of a risk is known as the "willingness to pay" principle which estimates how much people would be willing to pay to avoid it. Such estimates can be obtained by a number of indirect or direct methods. The cost of insurance policies provides an example.

Public debates about risk are fraught with difficulties. It is now widely accepted that the best option is full disclosure of the risks and comprehensive communication of associated information. This has been fully acknowledged by the Chief Medical Officer for England and Wales, who has proposed a system for standardising the terminology used in communicating risks.[100] The final acceptance of the risk may then depend on people's confidence in the risk management procedures that are proposed.

5.   *Submission and appraisal of the EIS*

5.1   Submission

The EIS is submitted to the competent decision-making authority. For projects coming under the remit of the Town and Country Planning (Assessment of Environmental Effects) Regulations 1988[101] in England and Wales, the competent authority is the Local Planning Authority. The inclusion of a non-technical summary improves the accessibility of information to the public. Although it is a requirement of the legislation to include such summaries, they are often omitted. The competent authority uses the EIS and any supporting information to determine whether or not planning consent should be granted, in the light of any possible adverse effects on the environment (including effects on human beings and their health).

The planning authority is normally required to determine planning applications subject to EIA within 16 weeks. Where the planning authority considers that the information provided in the EIS, together with that available to the authority from other sources, is inadequate to "permit proper evaluation of the project's likely environmental effects", the authority has the power to require the provision of further information. However, these powers are not exercised frequently, often due to limited resources, but sometimes due to a lack of expertise in appraising EISs. There is also a reluctance to 'clog up' the planning process by introducing further delays.

In the case of the Highways Agency, the draft highway orders, the Inspector's report of proceedings at Public Inquiry, the EIS Report and the Environmental Statement, must go to the Secretary of State for the Department of the Environment, Transport and the Regions (DETR) who will then consider whether to grant planning consent. This information may be copied to the Department of Health, but is not supplied to them automatically. The decision may be challenged in the High Court within six weeks of the publication of the decision letter.

5.2   Appraisal

Appraisal of EISs and the EIA-studies carried out to produce them, is an important part of the decision-making process. EISs may be appraised by specially convened panels. General review criteria are available which can help decision-makers to assess the quality of EISs with respect to compliance with the legislation, accuracy of content and appropriateness of scope.[102] There are no such review criteria relating specifically to health issues. Review of EISs with respect to their coverage of health issues reveals considerable shortcomings (see Appendix 6). Health and social welfare specialists should be involved in EIA appraisal and represented on appraisal panels. There is a need for integration of environmental and health input at the appraisal stage.

Environmental assessment does not usually include occupational health and safety. This is regarded as a specialist topic, regulated in the UK by the Health and Safety Executive. Yet occupational health and safety must be central to health impact assessment. While those engaged in HIA cannot become specialists in all subjects, they need to be informed of the legislative and regulatory framework. Those responsible for appraisal and review of EISs need to ensure that occupational health and safety has been duly considered in the planning application. The EIS should be appraised against the Terms of Reference. Consequently, if the requirements for HIA are properly addressed in the Terms of Reference this will be reflected in the amount of text in the report for a health specialist to appraise. Some of the text will be well supported by data and some will be based on assumptions. The health specialist should be able to exercise expert judgement about the conclusions that have been reached in the EIS.

There are still very few members of the public health or environmental health community who are trained and informed about the EIA process, and therefore poorly prepared for appraising EISs. There is a risk that the specialist recruited for the task will be a doctor whose expertise lies within clinical health care. Such a person may be unfamiliar with planning procedures outside the health service or with the technology used by the project developer or with the concerns of environmental and public health. Currently, the local Directors of Public Health, public health physicians and environmental health officers may prove not only important consultees in compiling the EIS, but may also have a role to play in appraising the EIS once it has been prepared by the consultant and submitted to the competent authority (ie the body from which consent must be obtained before the project can proceed). Consideration should be given to developing a specialty within public health related to environmental issues. Occupational health physicians, whose responsibilities include giving advice about the health aspects of the working environment (see Appendix 2), may also be able to provide a valuable source of expertise on the appraisal panel to address the health risks from industrial developments.

Decisions on the acceptability and management of the risks of exposure to hazardous agents identified by the EIA therefore require skill in interpreting toxicological and epidemiological data. Whilst public health physicians receive some training in toxicology and epidemiology, they may not have sufficient specialist expertise in human toxicology. They may lack comprehensive knowledge about the effects of all agents on all biological systems, since the range of information is enormous and incomplete. To participate most effectively on appraisal panels, public health physicians should have a familiarity with the essential steps in the assessment of risk, outlined above, and should receive training, including continuing education in all specialities related to environmental toxicology and environmental health.[103]

Environmental monitoring has been devolved to public health medicine following the report of the Abrams Committee in 1993[104] and as a branch of the profession used to multidisciplinary, multi-agency collaborative work, it may be possible for public health physicians to provide a liaison role, between toxicologists, epidemiologists and the planning authority in relation to the appraisal and subsequent management of the health risks of proposed development projects.

6. Negotiation and risk management

6.1 Negotiation

The final step before the decision is made on whether to allow the project to be implemented, is a process of negotiation between the major stakeholders in which the many costs and benefits of the project are collated and juxtaposed. Health impact assessment provides the negotiator with some of the tools needed for use in those negotiations. This is essentially a political rather than advisory matter and depends on many social priorities. It is important to stress that considerations of human health alone cannot determine whether a project is approved. To require otherwise would be to place health and health specialists apart from, and at the summit of, the decision-making ladder. This, in turn, could bring health impact assessment into disrepute as project proponents would resist participation in the assessment process. The negotiator's main objective should be to ensure that a budget for health mitigation is included in the project budget and that steps are taken to implement the mitigation measures that are agreed.

6.2 Health risk management

When it is concluded that a health risk may increase as a result of the policy, programme or project, health risk management strategies will be required. This is the third and final objective to be achieved by the process of incorporating health into EIA, namely:

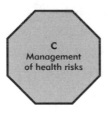

The preparation of action plans to mitigate negative impacts is a standard component of EIA and part of the Terms of Reference for external consultants.

The objective of health risk management is safeguarding health, mitigating health risks and seeking opportunities to improve health. It is essentially a preventative requirement, although curative measures will also be needed as a last resort. Human health is best safeguarded by modifications to project plans, operations and maintenance schedules. In some cases this can be achieved without substantial additional cost to the project: measures which improve the profitability of the project may simultaneously safeguard health. In other cases, early action would have prevented future costly litigation settlements, such as with asbestos, or sales reductions due to loss of confidence in the product. In other cases a percentage of total project cost must be allocated to this budget line. In the absence of a reliable economic valuation of impacts, a percentage of project cost should be reserved for safeguarding health in all projects. Alternative health safeguards could then be costed within that budget limitation.

There are many health risk management measures and they can be grouped according to whether they place responsibility on the individual or the society. In many cases a society component is required to balance that of the individual. For example, avoidance of traffic injury is not only the responsibility of the driver; the need for safer vehicles is widely accepted. In developing countries shortage of resources sometimes dictates a transfer of responsibility from society to the individual: malaria control has shifted from mass spraying to individual use of bednets; single disease control programmes have been replaced by horizontal approaches that depend on the support of local communities. The horizontal approach incorporates control of particular diseases into the activities of general health workers and redeploys specialised units to more general functions. Experience suggests that passive measures that do not require the active and continued co-operation of the community are more efficacious, but these must be included in project plans. Infrastructure that prevents the accumulation of waste water and contact with contaminated water, traffic regulators, pollutant emission controls and new agro-chemical formulations are all examples of passive measures that can be incorporated in project design and operation.

6.2.1   Risk management techniques

Risk management techniques employed at societal level include the following:

- Avoiding or eliminating the risk by prohibiting the use of a substance or activity, such as by zoning;

- Regulating the use of materials so as to reduce adverse health effects, such as control of chemical imports;
- Reducing vulnerability of people by using personal protective devices, such as helmets, masks, gloves and boots;
- Developing mitigation and recovery procedures after the event, such as emergency services and medical care;
- Instituting schemes to reimburse and redistribute losses, such as insurance.

In order to be effective, health risk management measures must also be socially acceptable to various sections of the community, reasonably costed and expected to be effective. The agencies responsible for implementation must be specified and the capacity of these agencies should be sufficient to undertake the task.

The following example of these risk management strategies is specific to road traffic injuries:

- Preventing the creation of the hazard by modifying the project design, eg by diminishing or preventing road traffic;
- Reducing the scale of particular hazards, eg by imposing speed limits;
- Preventing the creation of an existing hazard, eq by proper maintenance of machinery;
- Modifying the rate and distribution of release of the hazard, eg by using safety belts;
- Separating the hazard from the potential victims, eg by providing separate cycle ways;
- Separating the hazard and the potential victims by a barrier, eg traffic islands;
- Modifying the basic qualities of the hazard, eg make interior surfaces of vehicles crash absorbent;
- Make the human more resilient to the hazard, eg improved general health;
- Immediately counter the damage done, eg by providing first aid and rapid emergency response vehicles;

- Stabilise, repair and rehabilitate, eg by providing prompt and appropriate medical treatment and disability care.

Table 4: Health risk management example: occupational injury

	Vulnerability of community group	Environmental factors determining exposure to the hazard	Capacity and capability of health protection agencies
Pre-event	Behaviour modification to improve hazard avoidance	Separate community from hazard, by using barriers	Improve supervision and maintenance
Event	Employ people who are least vulnerable	Provide automatic shutoffs or speed regulators	Provide alarms for others to operate, such as emergency telephones
Post-event	Training people how to behave when injury occurs	Emergency machine release or emergency exits	Provide effective emergency services, subsequent care and rehabilitation

An alternative presentation of some risk management principles uses a matrix. The example given in Table 4 is concerned with occupational injury and is modified from Haddon.[105] It refers to the measures that may be taken before, during and after an injury event as part of risk management and is sub-divided according to the three essential components of health impact assessment referred to above.

In the case of hazardous substances, mitigation may involve:

- controlling emissions by pollution control, discharge reduction, recycling and reuse, substitution, reformulation, good housekeeping, reclamation or treatment;
- controlling movement by physical barriers such as clay liners in waste disposal sites and improved ventilation in work places.

However, some mitigation measures merely defer the risk and do not eliminate it. Examples include the containment facilities used for hazardous waste disposal, such as clay liners and vitrification of radioactive waste.

Mitigation is also likely to involve improvements in health-care facilities, occupational health services, emergency response plans, counselling, health education and 'lifestyle programmes'.[106] Vague suggestions for increased health education frequently occur in environmental assessments, but they have no value unless the resources, agenda, acceptability, educational materials and means of evaluation are specified in some detail.

7. *Monitoring and surveillance*

The EIA legislation emphasises the importance of taking appropriate mitigation measures to avoid, remedy or reduce any significant adverse impacts which are identified. There is, however, no formal requirement for monitoring the impacts attributable to a project once development consent has been granted. This makes it very difficult to establish whether proposed mitigation measures are either implemented or effective. Once planning permission has been obtained for a project, the planning authorities have little power to ensure that mitigation measures are implemented in their entirety unless they stipulate them as a condition on planning consent. All projects with potential adverse effects require recommendations for post-project activities. These may include monitoring and epidemiological surveillance, establishing advisory committees and notification mechanisms in case of malfunction. Local authorities should specify that developers earmark specific resources to ensure that such post-project activities take place. Such monitoring and surveillance would enable the local authority to establish whether the proposed mitigation measures had been effective, and identify any previously unforeseen risks or benefits associated with the project.

The Department of the Environment, Transport and the Regions in collaboration with the Department of Health should review the outcome of any mitigation measures and follow-on assessment. The information gained from such a review should be used to improve the design, methodology and conduct of future environmental impact assessments and health impact assessments, and to circulate guidance and disseminate guidelines on best practice, based on past experience.

In 1997, the DETR commissioned a study of the treatment of mitigation within EIAs.[107] The research found that:

- Of the 100 environmental impact statements reviewed, none were excellent in their treatment of mitigation, 18 were good, just over half were fair and almost a third were poor or worse;
- There was no detectable trend of improvement between 1990 and 1995 and few distinctions could be drawn between different types of projects.

In particular:

- The range of mitigation options considered was fairly restricted (for example, alternatives were not considered where they might have been, and there was attention on physical measures rather than on operational or management controls).
- Descriptions of mitigation were often imprecise and the status of undertakings was unclear.
- Little attention was paid to residual impacts after mitigation.

As a result of the study, the DETR plan to publish a 'Good Practice Guide' to encourage the consideration of mitigation in the project design process, and explain how mitigation should be treated in environmental impact statements.[108]

In order to develop methodology and learn from past assessments, the outcome of this monitoring, surveillance and other post-project activities should be reviewed as part of a periodic follow-on assessment. This should be undertaken for every project requiring an EIA or HIA, after an appropriate period, for example five years. Specific funding from the development project should also be set aside for this.

7.1   Monitoring

Monitoring is often contrasted with surveillance. Monitoring typically involves, for example, the measuring and recording of physical, social and economic variables associated with the development impacts (eg traffic flows, air quality, noise, employment level), in order to make management decisions during the implementation of a project. Surveillance, on the other hand, is a more routine process which collects information, eg on a specific health risk that may contribute to future decisions and evaluations. However, it should be noted that these terms may be used differently by professionals, such as those in the health care sector and environmental protection agencies.

Monitoring is important to the impact assessment process because it can assist regulatory authorities to:

- determine if mitigation measures have been implemented,
- provide a real-time understanding of a project's effects on health and well-being,
- resolve uncertainties,
- verify the accuracy of the assessment, and
- identify effects that were not anticipated.

A proposal for monitoring[109] should achieve the following:

- identify the roles, responsibilities and accountability of different stakeholders;
- specify the indicators to be monitored with frequency and location;
- specify the statistical methods to be used to analyse the results;
- outline how the results will be communicated and to whom.

The Environment Agency should devise effective monitoring systems, based on research to be undertaken by the Research Councils and appropriate government departments, to ensure that during implementation, projects and policies comply with the health risk management measures that have been agreed and that mitigation measures are effective.

7.2   Surveillance

Uncertainty is a seminal component of health impact assessment. Consequently, the health status of vulnerable communities may require regular surveillance during the implementation and operational phases of the project. This will often involve the use of indirect indicators of health and might be undertaken as an element of governmental provision within a national health impact assessment framework. As such, it could be a function of existing agencies such as the Department of Health's Central Health Monitoring Unit and its other UK counterparts.

Future needs of HIA

Gaining appropriate health information for future HIA

The review of EISs undertaken for this report (Appendix 6) identified a lack of clear procedures or methodologies for assessing health implications as a possible reason for the current lack of attention to human health issues. Statistical associations with risk factors cannot be determined with any certainty and remain speculative. However, epidemiology may provide a good method for analysing some of the health impacts of existing projects and this would strengthen the case for the health impact assessment of new projects. Obvious limitations include the difficulties of analysing multiple causes of health outcomes such as exposure to a cocktail of hazardous substances at low levels in the air we breathe and the water we drink. A systematic analysis of existing projects will be required to develop an appropriate database. This is an evaluation activity that feeds back data into the assessment process and has a time lag of 5-10 years. Analytical epidemiology cannot be used to predict the health risks of projects that have not yet been built except in the qualitative sense of arguing by analogy. Mathematical epidemiology based on models can be used for some health risks but there are great uncertainties and many assumptions have to be made. Such models usually have two main components: a function that distributes the dose of the hazardous agent between people ('exposure scenario') and a dose-response function.

In many cases the health impacts of a project are indirect and they may occur under conditions where many changes are taking place that are unrelated to the project.

The consequent environmental 'noise' may mean that statistical associations with risk factors cannot be determined with any certainty and remain speculative.

Development of health indicators

It is frequently difficult to measure changes in health directly and health indicators will be required as indirect and surrogate measures of those impacts. A wide range of different kinds of information may contribute to the development of those indicators. That could, for example, include various types of scientific information, as well as information about the beliefs and concerns of the public, especially forms of traditional knowledge held by people working in specific occupations.[110] Some characteristics of health indicators are that they must be:

- relevant to the possible health effects of the project,
- understandable by all stakeholders,
- capable of distinguishing between positive and negative health consequences, and
- quantifiable where possible.

Health indicators are likely to play an important role in the development of quantitative methods for HIA. Research is needed in the development of suitable indicators. Surrogate indicators must always be related back to the unmeasurable concept for which they are a proxy. Direct health indicators must only represent information which is conceptually quantifiable. Indicators must not be misused, for example to hide problems, to make policies look more or less successful, or to manipulate public debate.[111]

In proposing 'environment' as a key area in the *Health of the Nation* strategy,[112] the Government noted that in order to achieve improvements in health, the existing key areas in the *Health of the Nation* strategy should focus, in many cases, on specific health outcomes such as reduced incidence of coronary heart disease or cancers. In relation to the environment, however, the government recognised that:

- it is difficult to quantify and correlate direct health benefits with measures taken to improve the environment, due to confounding factors such as genetic predisposition, vulnerability to infection, stress, diet and lifestyle;

- as a result, improvements in environmental health cannot generally be measured as health outcomes — instead they are better measured in terms of health risks or potential causes of ill-health, such as dangerous levels of water or air pollution.

In some areas the Government proposed surrogate health indicators, eg the satisfactory resolution of domestic noise complaints to local authorities as a surrogate indicator of the success of measures to minimise noise pollution. The quantification of environmental impacts on health is not explicitly addressed in the recent document *Our Healthier Nation*,[113] and health indicators by which to measure environmental health targets are lacking.

Research methodology for HIA

Research on health impact assessment methodology cannot be carried out in a vacuum however, at present there are no groups of researchers in the UK specifically funded to undertake research into health impact assessment. A systematic and comprehensive programme of research is required to develop the methodologies with which HIA can be conducted. A variety of different bodies should be expected to contribute to this programme of research and a consortium should be established to fund, commission and direct that research. The membership of that consortium should include the Department of the Environment, Transport and the Regions, the Department of Health, the Natural Environment Research Council, the Medical Research Council, the Biotechnology and Biological Sciences Research Council, the Economic and Social Research Council, the Environment Agency and the Royal Commission on Environmental Pollution. The programme of work should be conducted by research teams comprising a diverse range of specialists, including health economists and those from the natural, medical and social sciences.

In order to develop a structure for strategic and project-level health impact assessment methodologies, a systematic review of the health hazards associated with a series of programmes, policies and projects in each sector should be conducted to assess their health risks. The development of methodologies for health impact assessment should ideally begin at the strategic level of policies, programmes and plans. The structured approach developed at strategic level should then be retained in developing project-level methodologies, which will take account of the practical levels of information available at the different levels.

In addition to research into the operation of the impact assessment process, discussed below, the research should focus on methods for generating the necessary data for use in impact assessments. A systematic review of the health hazards associated with developments in each sector should be carried out in order to produce a comprehensive checklist which could be used to guide developers and planning authorities. Hazards both directly and indirectly associated with the development should be included in the checklist. The importance of each hazard should be determined according to its frequency and severity. The checklist should also include sociological factors and perceived hazards for which there is little or no evidence, but high public concern.

There is an urgent need for much more epidemiological surveillance both of occupationally exposed groups and of the general population. The case for more systematic epidemiology starting from, but extending beyond, occupational settings has repeatedly been emphasised by the BMA. Occupational settings have the methodological advantage that people are often exposed in the course of their employment to relatively high concentrations of potentially hazardous materials and activities, and for relatively long periods of time. Consequently a thorough scrutiny of occupational settings can provide early warning signs of hazards to which the broader population may in due course also be exposed. Occupation and general epidemiology will also be important both for the conduct of HIAs and for research into ways of improving the methodologies of HIAs by providing baseline data sets against which the impact of proposed changes may be assessed.

The difficulties in extrapolating between the results of toxicity tests performed under laboratory conditions on animals, and estimates of likely effects on people, mean that adequate data required to carry out human health impact assessment are often seriously lacking. Laboratory and bench research is therefore required, with particular consideration given to:

- the development of new markers for monitoring and surveillance of health impact;
- improved estimates of exposure both for individuals and populations;

- better methods for extrapolating risk to populations, together with the ecological basis for risk assessment;
- exposure to, and effects of, mixtures of chemicals.

Operational research

Research is also needed into the operation of the assessment process. There should be an ongoing analysis of case studies of existing HIAs in order to identify good practice, to further develop concepts and provide models for future health impact assessments to follow. Such studies could usefully include a systematic review of UK planning applications to determine the extent to which human health is currently being addressed within the planning process, but also to clarify the relationship between planning procedures, inquiries and the conduct of HIAs within the EIA process. This work would help to define the boundaries within which a health impact assessment should be carried out.

Specific operational research should address the following:

- The way in which decisions are made at the screening stage to determine whether a project, policy, programme or plan requires an environmental health impact assessment to be carried out.
- At the scoping stage, how decisions are made regarding the health issues to be assessed.
- How the terms of reference are prepared and what they should contain.
- The appointment of expert advisers, eg as statutory consultees, or on the EIS appraisal panel.
- Risk management measures and the process by which these are agreed.
- Monitoring implementation of the project or policy etc and the effectiveness of mitigation measures.
- Post-project/policy follow-on studies.
- Requirements for adequate consultation which takes place at an early stage and continues throughout the assessment process.
- How committees, agencies and other bodies from different sectors, such as health care and environmental protection, could cooperate more effectively.

Examples of possible health impacts of UK projects

There is a range of possible linkages between projects and health in the UK context and some examples are given in Table 5. Transport is responsible for noise, injuries and deaths resulting from road traffic accidents and air pollutants that contribute to lung diseases.[114] Miners are especially at risk of injury and lung disease. The burning of fossil fuels in the energy sector contributes to air pollution and lung disease, while injury is associated with the use of heavy machinery and transport of fuel. Agriculture, including livestock

Table 5:
Examples of health/sector linkages

Sector	Communicable diseases	Non-communicable diseases	Inappropriate nutrition	Injury	Mental disorders
Transport	X	X		X	X
Mining	X	X		X	X
Energy		X		X	
Agriculture	X	X		X	
Fisheries				X	
Manufacture	X	X		X	X
Construction in general	X	X		X	
Tourism	X			X	
Food industry	X	X	X		
Housing	X	X			X

production, is associated with zoonoses, agro-chemical poisoning, and injuries from machinery such as tractors and binders and from many other sources. Deep-sea fishery workers are exposed to the risk of drowning. Manufacturing industry is associated with communicable disease where there are food products, occupational diseases such as dust induced lung disease, as well as injuries and deafness associated with heavy machinery. The production and consumption of inappropriate foods gives rise to many forms of dietary problems including obesity, hypertension, dental caries and diabetes. Tourism contributes to the promotion of sexually transmitted diseases and other infections. Mental disorders, including psycho-social problems, seem to be a facet of modern industrial life, including the excessive demands of the workplace.

The following examples illustrate some of the possible health impacts associated with airport development, industrial pollution, housing and indoor air quality, and occupation.

Example: Manchester Airport inquiry

Possibly the only example of a completed prospective health impact assessment in the UK is the (unpublished) submission to the Public Inquiry into the proposed second runway at Manchester Airport.[115] This illustrates the transport-health linkages identified in Table 5. A model was developed which estimated both positive and negative health effects of the predicted environmental changes consequent upon the development. The outcome was a report, based primarily on qualitative data, which emerged as a powerful negotiating tool at the Inquiry, where it contributed substantially to the mitigation package agreed between the Airport Authority and the Health Authorities concerned.

The process began with a multidisciplinary seminar where health service, environmental health and planning staff identified possible health impacts of various fictional planning proposals. These were then collated and the quantifiability of their impact was estimated, on a scale from 'speculative' to 'calculable'. Matrices showing the environmental and health impacts of major aspects of the proposal were then constructed, using the assumptions in the airport's environmental impact statement, and working with colleagues from additional disciplines such as geography, meteorology and toxicology. Although many of the predicted impacts could not be quantified, their identification alone

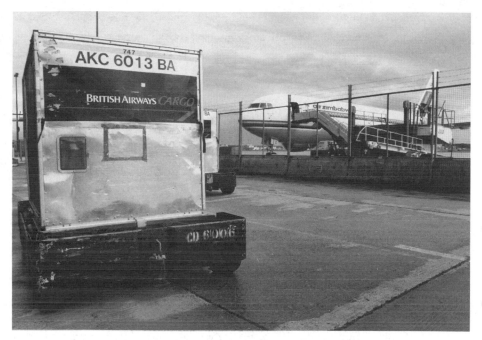

For the proposed development of a second runway at Manchester Airport, both positive and negative health effects were considered

raised sufficient concern for the report's recommendations to be largely accepted by the airport's planners.

Example: Industrial pollution

Much of the evidence considered in prospective assessments of this sort will inevitably originate from retrospective evaluations of existing hazards. A UK example of the complexity of such evaluations comes from the Teesside Environmental Epidemiology Study Group,[116] which examined the higher mortality of the population of disadvantaged areas of Teesside by comparison with similar areas of Sunderland. The major focus of the research was on the possible role of industrial air pollution. In addition to wide-ranging analyses of routinely collected health and demographic data, special studies were undertaken of air quality, general practitioner records, respiratory diseases and risk factors in the community. The work suggested that historical industrial emissions were likely to have contributed to increased levels of lung cancer. Although hypotheses concerning contemporary health impacts of industry could not be verified, the role of such studies in responding to legitimate public concern regarding health impacts should not be overlooked.[117]

Example: Housing and indoor air quality

Indoor air quality is a continuing problem in the UK, particularly as improved insulation and draft exclusion have reduced the rate at which air in the room is replaced. The indoor burning of various heating and cooking fuels can generate a wide range of pollutants. The indoor air pollutants posing the greatest hazard include carbon monoxide (100 accidental deaths per year), radon (a natural gas that seeps out of the ground) and environmental tobacco smoke (the latter two are associated with cancer). Also of concern are nitrogen dioxide (from gas cookers), house dust mites, and volatile organic compounds (all of which are implicated in the incidence of respiratory disease, especially in children), fungi, bacteria, and asbestos.[118] Poor indoor ventilation may lead to an increased risk of respiratory infections.[119,120]

A study of indoor air quality by the Building Research Establishment provided information on the range and concentration of pollutants occurring in typical family homes.[121] The main health hazards identified were the possible association between respiratory disease and exposure to nitrogen dioxide arising from gas cookers, and between asthma and exposure to house dust mites. Concerns were also expressed about the effect of formaldehyde (found in adhesives, disinfectants, textiles, photographic film, cosmetics and some wall insulation), and volatile organic compound levels (arising from painting and decorating). WHO exposure thresholds for all these substances were exceeded in a proportion of the homes examined. Mitigation measures could include a policy of requiring low-emission standards in all new products.[122]

Radon gas is found quite naturally in rock and soil, but it is also present in building materials such as bricks and can seep into the indoor air of a building, and therefore needs to be controlled by adequate ventilation. In Britain, a wide variety of indoor radon concentrations have been found depending on the rate of ventilation and how and where the buildings have been built. In general, the highest concentration of radon has been found in Devon and Cornwall, with the average dose in Cornwall being three times higher than the UK average. Figures from the National Radiological Protection Board suggest that radon exposure in the UK could be responsible for approximately 2,500 lung cancer deaths per year.[123]

The BMA welcomed the government's proposal to incorporate the environment as a key area within the *Health of the Nation* strategy and to include targets for air quality in homes.[124] In the 1998 revision *Our Healthier Nation*,[125] indoor air quality remains an area of concern, but this focuses mainly on indoor air pollution caused by smoking in the home and the workplace. In order to demonstrate its full commitment to improving indoor air quality, the government should ban all forms of tobacco advertising. The problem of radon in the home is mentioned in relation to cancer prevention. Unless the strategy, *Our Healthier Nation*, is extended to include other factors of indoor air quality, it will fail to address the environmental and health consequences of poor air quality at work or in public buildings, where people may spend a large proportion of time. The 1994 BMA report *Environmental and Occupational Risks of Health Care*[126] identified the need for improved control of waste anaesthetic gases in the work place. Other issues covered included building design and sick building syndrome, exposure to fumes from formaldehyde and other chemicals in the workplace.

The BMA Board of Science and Education has highlighted the correlation between poor housing and ill health in an 'occasional paper'.[127] Although the provision of information on the health effects of key indoor pollutants is important, the opportunity for individuals to make positive choices about indoor air quality may not be available to those on low income. The BMA recommended the "building and refurbishment of more homes for rent, at an affordable cost and renewal of housing stock".[128] In addition, consideration should be given to providing financial assistance for improving indoor air quality to particularly vulnerable groups.

Example: Occupation

It has been estimated that the overall cost of work-related ill health and accidents is between £.11-16 billion every year or 2-3% of Gross Domestic Product (GDP).[129] Occupational injury risks are highest in the energy and water supply sector, followed by

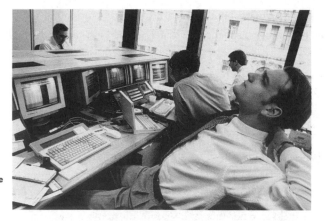

construction, agriculture, forestry and fishing. Deep sea fishing and offshore oil and gas work are particularly high risk occupations.

Occupationally related psychiatric disorder and stress may also have a high cost to industry. One USA source has estimated the costs of stress and stress compensation claims in terms of absenteeism, lost productivity, retraining and health care to be up to $150 billion per year.[130] Hurrell noted that compensation claims for occupational stress-related illnesses were the fastest growing type of claim in the 1980s, comprising more than 11% of all worker compensation claims.[131] In 1992, the BMA published *Stress and the medical profession*[132] which drew attention to the high levels of suicide, alcoholism and drug abuse among doctors.

Occupational stress may have a high cost to industry

In a further report on the misuse of alcohol and other drugs by doctors,[133] the BMA noted that two thirds of all cases referred to the GMC health procedures involved the misuse of alcohol and other drugs, and estimated that one in 15 doctors in the UK may suffer from some form of dependence. The report made a number of recommendations to address the problem, including provision of access to a comprehensive occupational health service and the need for research to inform policy makers when taking strategic decisions on service development. The report concluded that instances continue to occur where impairment of doctors through alcohol and other drug misuse constitutes a threat to patient welfare. In order to address public concern, the medical profession must monitor progress and modify policies in relation to this issue.

As another example, the Chief Medical Officer estimated in 1994 that up to 1.5 million workers are exposed to hazardous noise, and surveys in the 1980s indicated that 52,500 people were affected by occupational deafness in England and Wales.[134]

Examples of the health impacts of UK policy

There is an enormous variety of public policies that have implications for the environment and health.[135] These range from direct environmental policies, such as those relating to transport, or to social and economic policies — for instance, the imposition of Value Added Tax on fuel or the introduction of water metering.

Recent guidelines from Canada provide additional examples of the behavioural and socio-economic changes associated with policies that could have a health impact.[136] These are summarised in Table 6.

Table 6: Some associations between policy and health

Type of policy	Some behavioural and socio-economic changes with potential health impact
Macroeconomic	● Income distribution and level; ● Changes in labour market; ● Changes in cost of living, food and housing; ● Effects on health sector.
Agriculture	● Effect of agricultural subsidies on pesticide use and residues, food production, farm income and rural way of life.
Industrial	● Use and promotion of toxic substances; ● Requirements for pollution control; ● Hazardous waste regulation; ● Occupational health and safety requirements; ● Liability for remedial action and clean-up.
Energy	● Nuclear fuel cycle; ● Effects of "smog"; ● Global warming.
Housing and social	● Overcrowding; ● Access to safe water; ● Adequate waste collection and treatment; ● Indoor air quality.
Natural resources	● Migration; ● Resettlement.

Table 7: Examples of health/policy linkages

Policy	Communicable diseases	Non-communicable diseases	Inappropriate nutrition	Injury	Mental disorders
VAT on fuel	✘	✘	✘		
Full fat milk subsidies		✘	✘		
Road transport		✘		✘	✘
Nuclear energy		✘		✘	
Water metering	✘				
Housing	✘	✘		✘	✘
Out-of-town shopping		✘	✘	✘	✘

There is a need to develop and to test methods for undertaking prospective assessment of these policies. Table 7 illustrates some of the possible linkages, a selection of which are discussed in the examples that follow.

Example: VAT on domestic fuel

A retrospective assessment of the health impact of the introduction in 1994 of Value Added Tax on domestic fuel may not be easy to conduct. However, previous research on fuel poverty permitted the prospective judgement that the effects would stem from reduced disposable incomes of those vulnerable groups with no choice but to pay the increased prices.[137] These effects would include a reduction in resistance to infection and cardiovascular disease, morale and efficiency among pensioners, and low income families with young children. Secondary effects on the affordability of good quality food could also be predicted.

Example: Transport policy

The current transport system and planning policy has led to more people becoming dependent on the motor car, making the environment more hostile for others, even including those in motor cars. Car ownership has risen from 5.7 million in 1960 to around 23 million in 1995.[138] Private transport externalises a range of consequences so that the individual is effectively asking society as a whole to pay for their car usage; this is neither cost-effective nor environmentally sustainable; nor is it beneficial to human health.

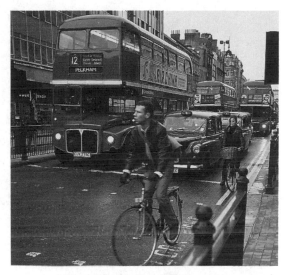

The current hostile traffic environment may have a detrimental effect on the use of health promoting forms of transport such as cycling

Transport policy can influence health in a number of ways. Road traffic accidents and air pollution are the obvious effects and are the easiest to measure — in 1996, 44,473 people were reported seriously injured and 3,598 were killed on roads in the UK[139] and air pollution has been linked to increases in asthma and chronic respiratory symptoms.[140,141] There can be other negative, more indirect effects of transport policy on health such as:

- noise pollution from traffic, which is known to affect sleep and mental health and may have important psycho-social effects with evidence for depression amongst people exposed to high levels of traffic noise.[142] It is also accepted that long term exposure to traffic noise can result in noise induced hearing loss.[143] Traffic noise can reduce perceived environmental quality, increase sleeping problems and health worries which may lead to recourse to health services;[144]

- community severance, social support and neighbourhood quality, which can be indirectly influenced by transport policy. Low levels of social support have been linked to increased mortality rates from all causes[145] and a review of the role of psycho-social stress and social support concluded that both had an influence on coronary heart disease, but social support more so than stress.[146] The severance effect of motor traffic reduces access to social support networks and health promoting facilities for those travelling on foot or by bicycle, including shops and health facilities;

- personal safety fears, which appear to have increased significantly in recent years and have had a detrimental effect on the use of health promoting forms of transport such as walking or cycling. Busy roads can also be intimidating to pedestrians and they are more exposed to accidental injury, pollution, noise and stress. A perceived danger of travel can also cause feelings of anxiety. Children's freedom and independence has been curtailed because of this.[147] Low income households are more likely to be reliant on public transport and to have suffered most from the effects of bus-deregulation and a decline in public transport services. The elderly, children and people with disabilities are also particularly disadvantaged by current transport policies and may suffer increasing feelings of isolation and insecurity due to curtailment of their freedom and independence.

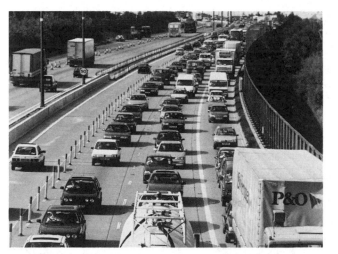

The health impact of transport infrastructure should be assessed alongside traditional methods of cost benefit analysis

Against this, the benefits of more health promoting forms of transport have been widely documented and it is accepted that increases in physical activity, (eg, walking and cycling) could significantly increase individual and public health. Physical activity has been shown to reduce the risk of coronary heart disease and stroke, obesity and hypertension. It has also been shown to increase self-esteem and confidence and to be an effective treatment for depression and anxiety.[148]

Demand is exceeding supply for road space, and measures to reduce the adverse impacts of cars (eg, emission controls) will be outweighed by demand. There is therefore a need to reduce demand and encourage a modal shift to other more health promoting forms of transport, such as cycling. It is accepted that it is neither environmentally acceptable nor economically viable to meet this demand. What needs to be recognised is that it is also not acceptable to public and individual health.

The BMA in its 1997 report, *Road Transport and Health*,[149] noted that examination of the health issues relating to transport enabled a number of policies to be proposed to reduce risk and promote health, including implementation of an integrated and sustainable public transport system. However, transport targets to promote health need to do more than just seek increases in travel by walking, cycling and public transport; national road traffic targets also need to be set to reduce car use.

The BMA recommended[150] that the Department of Health should contribute to the development of a health audit to assess the health impact of new transport infrastructure, which should be considered alongside traditional transport cost benefit analysis. Future planning policies for transport need not only to consider the economic effects on society, but also the consequences to the environment and human health which bring about their own indirect economic costs. The Government plans to publish a fundamental review of transport policy in 1998.

The Environment Agency has also begun to address the costs of road transport with the publication of an initial assessment of the environmental impact of road transport.[151] The publication considers both the present impact and the likely future effects of trends in vehicle use, and identified issues such as the exploitation of raw materials, accidents which cause pollution, and road building and maintenance, as important risks to the state of our environment. It acknowledged that future road transport options will need to ensure, as far as possible, that transport decisions reflect the true costs, by reducing the social and environmental impacts. From previous studies of the costs of environmental damage, such 'true' costs appear to be substantial. Table 8 illustrates the cost of some environmental impacts of private passenger road transport.

This initial assessment marks the start of a more in-depth study to look at the issues surrounding road transport, during which the Environment Agency plans to seek to quantify risks, to assess the relative merits of options to prevent environmental damage, and

Table 8:
Cost of environmental impacts of private road transport

Environmental impact	£ per 1000 passenger/kilometres	Approximate annual total cost, UK £ billion
Air pollution	4.3 (urban) 1.7 (other)	1.12[1] 0.52[1]
Air pollution (health effects)	14.0 (urban) 2.5 (all)	1.5[2]
Noise	1.8	1.0[2]
Water pollution	2.2	1.2[2]

[1] *Based on 190 billion kilometres driven on non-built up roads and 163 billion kilometres driven on built-up roads in 1995 and 1.6 passenger/car.*

[2] *Assuming 353 billion kilometres driven in 1995 and 1.6 passenger/car. Costs are taken from diverse sources and should not be summed, care should be taken in comparing between costs.*

to determine the economic impact of these measures. Such a study may provide valuable risk data for future impact assessments and should include examination of the health risks associated with transport policy.

Example: Water metering

In 1989 the BMA's Annual Representative Meeting expressed concern about the health impacts of the then forthcoming privatisation of the water supply industry. The matter was raised again in 1993, and in 1994 the BMA published a review of the health impacts of privatisation with particular focus on the effects of disconnections to domestic properties.[152] Key aspects of this study are given below.

Health hazard identification

In addition to social impact, the major health hazards associated with inadequate supplies of clean water in the UK were identified as hepatitis A and dysentery caused by *Shigella sonnei*. Both of these communicable diseases are known to exhibit cyclic epidemics in the UK and are spread by the faecal-oral route of transmission. A peak of the epidemic cycle occurred in the years immediately after privatisation when disconnections were significantly increased, and the peak prevalence rate appeared to be higher than in the recent past.[153]

Community vulnerability

People who are particularly vulnerable to shortages of clean water include the very young, the very old and the disabled, who have difficulty in cleaning themselves properly after defecation and urination. Other groups include those with medical conditions that require frequent bathing, such as eczema and psoriasis sufferers, or who need water for treatment such as renal dialysis patients. Water is also needed to wash soiled clothing and bed linen of those who are suffering from acute diarrhoea, for example. People with very low incomes or suffering deprivation were considered to be particularly vulnerable.

Environmental factors

The BMA was principally concerned with the health effects of domestic disconnection and reductions in water use associated with metering, high water rates, indebtedness and attempts to reduce domestic consumption.

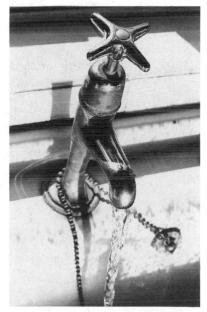

Capacity and capability of agencies involved

The report analysed the capability of Ofwat, the Office of Water Services, to regulate and monitor the water supply industry. It also analysed the behaviour of the 32 private water supply companies that were formed in England and Wales.

A great deal of inconsistency in methods and levels of charging for water between companies was found. The cost of water had risen sharply following privatisation. It has been estimated that about 22% of water put into distribution systems is lost before it reaches customers.[154] However, the cost of leakages is borne by consumers, as is the cost of the removal of pollution caused by agricultural chemicals.[155]

Clean water is vital to halting the chain of infection and should be available to all at an affordable price

There was poor provision of flexible methods of payment that would assist those on low incomes to budget for water use. The number of disconnections had increased sharply and there was great variability between companies. Those with water meters were paying considerably more for their water than those without.

Change in health risk attributable to the policy

The association between water supply and sanitation and communicable disease is fundamental to public health and was proved by the dramatic improvement in the public health during the nineteenth century. However, it can be very difficult to prove a causal link between a policy of water disconnection and ill-health. The general evidence is regarded as sufficient to invoke the precautionary principle: reductions in water use and disconnection due to financial hardship are likely to lead to an increased risk of communicable disease. Putting individual households at risk is likely to increase the risk to the general community with whom the household have contact. This conclusion is supported by recent research undertaken among low income families.[156]

Health risk management

The infectious diseases identified above can only be held in check by high standards of hygiene. Water is vital to halting the chain of infection and should be available to all at an affordable price.

The BMA made several recommendations, including the following:

- Disconnection of domestic water supply for reasons of non-payment should be made illegal;
- An equitable system for setting water charges should be established;
- Water companies should provide their customers with a flexible method of payment.

Example: Housing policy

One of the earliest examples of UK government housing policy which had poor health impacts must be the seventeenth century Window Tax that reduced light and ventilation to people's dwellings.[157] The 1960s policy of mass building using untried techniques produced homes that could not be kept warm and dry. Through-beams in slab block constructions act as cold bridges, reducing the effectiveness of insulating external walls; precast concrete slabs have a high thermal mass and rooms do not feel warm until the slabs have been heated.[158] Poor people can spend twice as much of their total income on heating compared to others. Although there are many confounding factors, such as family size and passive smoking, there may also be a dual influence of cold and damp living conditions on childhood respiratory disease.

One of the earlier studies of the effect of housing projects on health took place in 1933 in Stockton-on-Tees.[159] A community of slum dwellers were moved into a new housing project. A study of the children of the slum households reported that the infant mortality rate increased and nutritional status declined. These increases in health risk were believed to have arisen because the physical surroundings of the slum dwellers had improved, but household budgets had shifted away from spending on food because the community could not afford the increased rents of the new housing.

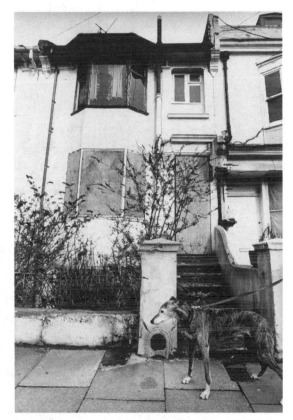

Poor housing may contribute to childhood respiratory disease and other health problems

Example: Asbestos

Since 1924, it had been appreciated that certain occupational health hazards were associated with asbestos, but the information was not appropriately communicated and surprisingly little action was taken to safeguard human health. The costs in both human suffering and economic loss are now being paid.

During the late 1920s legislation required improved ventilation in British asbestos factories. In the USA, knowledge about the hazard appears to have been deliberately suppressed by insurance companies and manufacturers throughout the 1930s and 1940s, according to some accounts.[160] During the 1940s, guidance on threshold dust levels was issued in the UK. In the USA alone, the use of asbestos increased 8-fold during the Second World War. Between 1938 and 1986 the permissible exposure limit in the USA was reduced by a factor of 150 times as the dose-response relationship and the range of associated diseases were better understood.[161] In 1964, a study of the hazard to insulation workers was published. In the late 1960s legislation enabled Americans to sue for compensation for the first time. There was evidence that workers had been deliberately misled and punitive damages were awarded. In 1978, it was estimated that 5.6 million Americans might die

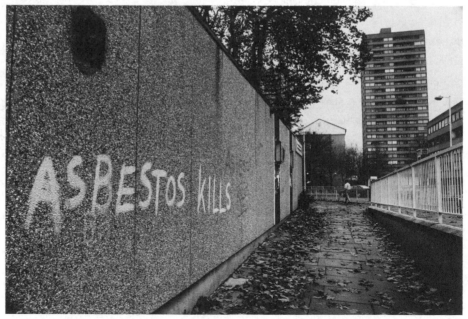

Asbestos-related diseases constitute the most serious single category of occupational disease

prematurely as a result of occupational exposure. In 1982, a leading manufacturer was bankrupted after paying hundreds of millions of dollars in compensation and legal costs. It has been estimated that the number of asbestos related compensation claims is likely to increase until 2010-2025 and to cost the insurance industry $50-100 billion; underwriters have been bankrupted and the market itself has been rocked.[162]

In 1997, it was estimated that there were approximately 3,500 deaths from asbestos exposure per annum in the UK. During 1996 there were, however, only five prosecutions under the Asbestos (Licensing) Regulations 1983, with an average fine of just £1,200 per conviction. There were also 21 convictions under the Control of Asbestos at Work Regulations 1987, with an average fine of £1,333.[163] Asbestos-related diseases constitute the most serious single category of occupational disease. Exposure to asbestos is associated with three asbestos-related diseases; asbestosis, mesothelioma and lung cancer. Asbestosis is a form of pulmonary fibrosis which is diagnosed by certain clinical features, presenting with a history of asbestos exposure and other signs such as pleural plaques. The only identified cause of mesothelioma is asbestos exposure, and the majority of cases now occurring can be assumed to be caused by asbestos exposure. There is a long latent period between first exposure to asbestos and the development of mesothelioma which is seldom less than 15 years and can be as long as 60 years. The disease is almost invariably fatal within one year of diagnosis. That most of this exposure is occupational in nature is suggested by the contrast between rates for men and for women, and by the high proportional mortality ratios recorded among occupations with a clear potential for substantial asbestos exposure. However, the wide range of occupations appearing on mesothelioma death certificates suggests that asbestos exposure sufficient to lead to mesothelioma is not confined to those occupational situations where asbestos exposure is routine or obvious.[164]

From 1969 to 1991, deaths due to mesothelioma have increased seven-fold for men and four-fold for women. There were a total of 1,009 deaths in 1991. Comparison of age specific rates in successive birth cohorts showed rates increasing steeply and continuously from the earliest cohorts, born at the end of the last century, up to the cohort born in the early 1940s. Rates for more recent birth cohorts are lower, by 30% for births around 1950, and by 40% for births around 1955. Despite these decreases, the number of deaths in these latest cohorts are still substantially above the levels seen for the earliest cohorts. Mortality follow-up of some 55,000 asbestos workers covered by the Health and Safety Executive asbestos worker survey showed an overall excess of 200 deaths from lung cancer, 183 from mesothelioma and 90 deaths involving asbestosis (in the absence of lung cancer or mesothelioma). These excesses were significantly more marked among those reporting their first exposure to asbestos as occurring before1970. When broken down by occupational sector, the highest excess mortality is seen in insulation workers, who had 33% excess mortality from lung cancer, mesothelioma and asbestosis combined. No other occupational sector approached this level of excess deaths.[165]

Exposure to asbestos contrasts with exposure to most other hazardous materials where associations between an adverse health effect and exposure to a substance are difficult or impossible to make with any degree of confidence, in an individual case, especially when the individual has been exposed to low levels over a long period of time.[166]

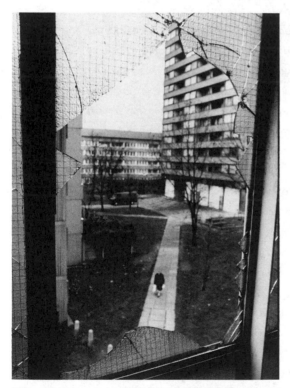

However, the stage has been set for future litigation and compensation claims. Perhaps the tobacco industry will be next in line. The cost of compensation may also stimulate industry to undertake health impact assessment to ensure that all reasonable precautions have been taken in advance.

Example: Out of town shopping

A 1987 planning enquiry into a Manchester out of town shopping centre included a presentation on health impacts.[167] This predicted: a reduction in the availability and an increase in the cost of healthy food in local shops; increased dependence on private cars and associated injuries; disruption of social support networks in deprived areas. The vulnerable groups were considered to be those already disadvantaged. The report cited evidence that poor people are

Vulnerable groups are most disadvantaged by reduction in availability and increase in cost of healthy food in local shops

often aware of what constitutes a healthy diet, but do not have access to or cannot afford healthy food. The enquiry noted that the risk of death from heart disease was 70% higher than average in the most deprived areas of the city. It also cited evidence that there is a close correlation between social support networks and physical health, and suggested that social support networks are often centred around local shopping centres in the inner city.

Example: Disaster planning

Health impact assessment is distinct from disaster planning, but there are many occasions when the assessment will need to be able to show that an adequate disaster plan has been formulated. Disaster plans often focus on the acute phase, ie warning people about the potential disaster and thus saving life. The chronic long term impacts that affect recovery and regeneration may not receive attention. For example, the consequences of the 1992 Los Angeles civil unrest included the following: 20 drug programme and alcohol recovery sites damaged, 15 health centres closed, 38 private medical and dental offices and 45 pharmacies damaged or destroyed, inspection of 2827 burned sites for asbestos hazards, 1000 food facilities damaged, 20% increase in landfill disposal for the following three months, 53 deaths, 2325 injuries, 248 hospital admissions, and an estimated $735 million damage.[168]

Example: Food policy

The issue of BSE (Bovine Spongiform Encephalopathy) has raised great concerns amongst the public about the safety of food and mistrust in government action in relation to food safety.

BSE was first identified as a disease in cattle in 1986 and was known to belong to a group of fatal diseases known as Transmissible Spongiform Encephalopathies which affect the brain. Much was, and still is, unknown about the infective agent (thought to be a prion protein), its transmission, and the implications for human health. In 1987, the Government claimed that the only route of transmission to cattle was from the use of scrapie infected (a spongiform disease found in sheep) animal remains being processed into cattle feed stuffs, and then infected cattle remains also being added to cattle feed. In

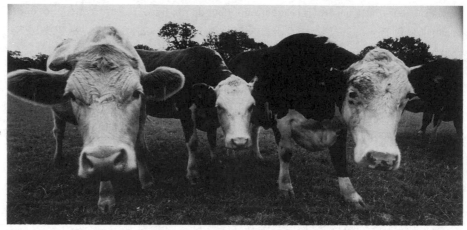

Concern over the possible link between BSE in cattle and CJD in humans led to a number of restrictions on meat production

1988 a series of bans preventing animal remains being used for cattle and sheep feed were introduced. Further bans were introduced in 1989 preventing specified bovine offal being used in human food. Unfortunately these bans were not strictly enforced and the number of BSE cases continued to rise. Most recently beef on the bone has been banned for human consumption, the direct public sale of which has been made illegal.

Much of the research into BSE has focused on the potential implications for human health and whether there is a link between BSE and Creutzfeldt-Jakob Disease (CJD) — a spongiform disease of the human brain leading to dementia and certain death. In March 1996, a new variant of CJD (nvCJD) was identified in ten cases, in people aged under 42 with dates of onset of illness in the previous two years. The government's Spongiform Encephalopathy Advisory Committee concluded that the possible cause of nvCJD was eating beef infected with BSE, but that a quantitative risk assessment could not provide an estimate of the absolute risk in relation to BSE. A precise measure was impossible because of the number of interacting uncertainties, including the long gestation period of the infection and the magnitude of the species barrier between cattle and man.[169] They advised that all restrictions on meat production should be strictly and fully implemented and that further research was required. By 31 January 1998 the total number of definite and probable cases of nvCJD was 23.[170]

The public demand for cheap food and the lack of effective regulation have been blamed as causes of the BSE/nvCJD crisis. However, international pressures to cut costs in agriculture, food production and distribution involving recycling animal wastes into animal feedstuffs have also played a part. Much of the focus of the BSE/nvCJD debate has been on consumer confidence in the meat industry rather than on the health of the public.

CHAPTER 5

Wider social and economic issues

The need for comprehensive health impact assessment

The current consensus that there are virtually no actions that do not impact on health has a long history; the first Medical Officer of Health was appointed in Liverpool in 1847 for precisely this reason. For much of the 20th century, however, the crucial dependence of public health on public policy has been eclipsed by an individualistic approach, stemming first from the germ theory of disease and later from the successes of immunisation and effective medical therapies.[1] Although there was renewed recognition of the broad range of health determinants two decades ago[2,3] it has taken many years for the implications of this understanding to be re-established. The World Health Organisation's *Health For All* strategy (1985) and a series of publications which commenced with the Black Report on Inequalities in health[4,5] have been particularly influential in this area. Now that the focus has shifted towards multisectoral actions to improve public health[6] there is a pressing need to find ways of evaluating such action. The aim should be to extend health impact assessment beyond its environmental project role to encompass the full range of policies, programmes and plans that can influence the public health.[7] What is ideally required are prospective methods that will enable the prediction of potential threats to health, so that action can be taken to ensure that negative outcomes are diminished or avoided.

Methodological guiding principles

While it is beyond the scope of this report to examine in detail the options for the new methods outlined above, some of the relevant issues are worthy of consideration. To summarise, in an ideal situation assessments would routinely be:

- multidisciplinary
- participatory
- equity-focused
- qualitative as well as quantitative
- multi-method
- explicit in their values and politics, and
- open to public scrutiny.

Multidisciplinary

Multidisciplinary assessments are required because the complexity of public health issues rarely, if ever, allows an assessment from the perspective of any one single discipline. Experience with environmental impact assessment (EIA) and with policy evaluation has shown that, irrespective of the skills of the expert assessor, there is added value in incorporating specialist — and generalist — inputs from the widest possible range of participants.

Participatory

A frequent criticism is that assessments are too narrowly technical and that those who will be, or have been, affected by the impact under consideration have not been involved in assessing its effects. Ideally the communities concerned should be full and equal participants in the assessment process. Among the benefits of this would be the increased chances of voluntary acceptance of risks by an informed community, as studies of risk perception suggest that voluntary risks are more acceptable than involuntary ones.[8]

Equity-focused

Health impact assessments should estimate the differential implications of the proposed actions for the various geographical, social class, gender, racial, age and other social groups affected. The Department of Health[9] has committed itself to action to reduce the widening inequalities in health in England. Equity in health is important not only because of its close relationship with social inequalities generally,[10] but also because it is frequently the most disadvantaged groups in the population who are affected first — and most — by health-damaging public policy. Assessments of the implications for the social and other dimensions of equity in health (eg gender, racial, age, geographical) are therefore of crucial importance.

Qualitative as well as quantitative

Requests for, and attempts to provide, quantitative assessments of cost and of health risk have understandably dominated debates about EIAs. As health impact assessment begins to extend across a broad range of public policies, qualitative methods will become equally important in obtaining a complete picture of the impacts studied. In methodological terms, this means that interviews and focus groups can bring out subtleties that quantitative surveys fail to pick up, or can explore in depth the individual experiences/opinions which are reflected in statistical data.

Multi-method

Ideally, a range of methods should be employed in each assessment. This is often called triangulation. The obvious advantage of this is that results from each method will tend to qualify each other's validity, where they cover overlapping issues.

Explicit values and politics

Values, ideologies and politics are unavoidable components of the assessment process[11,12] and values and interests should therefore be declared at an early stage by all participants. In addition to the values and politics of the participants themselves, the choice of different research methods may be rooted in the interests and values of particular investigators. For example, researchers may wish to focus on the collection and analysis of different types of information — and these decisions need to be acknowledged.

Public scrutiny

The purpose of health impact assessment is to contribute to the protection and maintenance of the public's health through the prevention or management of avoidable health hazards. It should therefore be an open process, undertaken in the full public gaze. This ideal may not always be achievable — for instance, where commercial secrecy applies — but it should nonetheless be an explicit aim. The public availability of information can provide companies that have poor environmental and health policies with incentives to act in accordance with the standards expected of so-called 'ethical investors'.

Links with social and other impact assessment

In addition to environment and health impact assessment, a number of other approaches exist which emerging methods for prospective HIA should consider. These include social impact assessment, policy evaluation and economic appraisal. These are all established methods within their own respective disciplines of EIA, applied economics, and policy analysis. This diversity indicates the importance of multidisciplinary approaches within HIA.

A form of analysis know as 'social impact assessment' (SIA) has been developed primarily within the USA, where it has been regarded as an integral element of EIA following the National Environmental Policy Act of 1969. It has also been applied in Australasia.[13] The guidelines and principles published in the US in 1994[14] set out a model which has many similarities to the stages of an EIA. However, the relative failure of SIA to make a difference in the project/policy decision process[15] suggests that current methods of SIA should not be uncritically imported into future models for HIA in the UK.

The consequences of ignoring health impact

It would be legitimate to raise the question of whether or not the costs of investing in developing methodologies and in pilot projects for prospective health impact assessments would exceed the likely benefits. One appropriate response to that line of inquiry might be to consider the implications of failing to act. The work of policy analysts and other recent research can indicate the probable costs of maintaining the status quo, and the benefits of taking action.

For instance, it is widely accepted that government's economic and social policies have resulted in substantial increases in poverty and in economic, social and health inequalities in the UK during the 1980s.[16,17,18] In some cases the resulting health damage has been quantified. Male unemployment causes three excess deaths annually for every 2000 unemployed men[19] and recent evidence[20] suggests that this level of excess mortality is continuing. In other cases, such as the examples given earlier relating to the imposition of volumetric water metering and of Value Added Tax on domestic fuel, the evidence of possible or actual health damage is chiefly qualitative and no less persuasive than quantitative research.

Additional areas where research suggests that undertaking and implementing the results of HIA is likely to yield net health benefits include the strengthening of the Health and Safety and Factory Inspectorates, the introduction of minimum nutritional standards for school meals, and the coordination of food safety with agricultural policy.

Health impact assessment and health economics

The difficulties of quantifying health impacts have been summarised in an earlier section of this report. One area where this has been partly addressed is in the field of health economics. In this section, we briefly review how the principles and methods of economics are being applied by health economists, and consider the relationship between the economic aspects of health and the design and conduct of health impact assessments.

Economics, health economics and concepts of efficiency

Economics is commonly defined as the study of how limited resources may be used to produce goods and services to meet human wants and needs. Health economics can tell an investigator how health care resources may be used to produce goods and services to meet human wants and needs for health care.[21] Health economists, like their colleagues in the broader economics profession, promote the concept of efficiency, the limitation of waste and the maximisation of measurable benefits to society from available resources. In the private sector, choices about resource use are guided by competitive markets.

Markets work by stimulating more production or reaching excess production. Markets are considered inefficient when:

- the buyer lacks the knowledge to decide what they need;
- social equity demands equal access to the product;
- catastrophic risk leads to widespread insurance;
- the costs of the production process fall on individuals;
- the production of a commodity cannot be increased to meet demand ('positional goods').

These last two points are of particular relevance to health impact assessment.

In the public sector, choices are more often guided by the question "What is best for society?" There is then the need for some technique to assess the relative net benefits of proposed investments from a societal perspective. One technique used by economists for this purpose is called 'cost-benefit analysis' (CBA), and it is a tool of economic evaluation. Cost-benefit analysis is a procedure for comparing the present value of some costs with the present value of the expected benefits for particular investments. CBA assumes that investments should be undertaken only if the present value of the benefits exceeds the present value of the costs.[22]

Cost-benefit analysis was first used in the UK to assess whether public investment in the M1 motorway should take place, ie whether or not the benefits of completing the project would outweigh the costs.[23] Comparison was made of the construction costs, plus the costs of compensating relocated families and businesses and the costs to the natural environment of damage, with the expected benefits from the improved mobility of people and goods such as increased employment. It was concluded that the benefits did indeed outweigh the costs and so the investment was approved. Since then CBA has been widely used in many EIAs.

Economists are concerned with identifying efficient ways of allocating scarce resources. Economists differentiate between two sorts of 'efficiency', namely what they refer to as 'allocative efficiency' and 'technical efficiency'. Allocative efficiency is achieved when the *maximum benefit is achieved from given resources*. Technical efficiency is maximised, on the other hand, when the *greatest possible output is obtained from a given quantity of inputs*, or a *given result is obtained from the minimum of resources*. CBA is based on the concept of allocative, rather than technical, efficiency because the analysis is designed to try to ensure that the benefits from new or continued investments are greater than the benefits which might accrue from deploying those resources elsewhere.

Ideally, cost-benefit analyses require that all costs and benefits, direct, indirect or intangible, be expressed in monetary units. However, the necessity and difficulty of having to value all costs and benefits in monetary terms has limited the extent to which the technique of cost-benefit analysis has been applied within the health sector. A central problem has been that it is extremely difficult to quantify health gains and health losses, and it is even more problematic to represent changes in mortality and morbidity in monetary terms.[24,25,26] Economists routinely use what is known as 'sensitivity analysis' to counteract the effects of the uncertainties in the quantification and monetisation of health impacts within CBAs. The investigators examine the consequences for the overall conclusion of the study, by varying some of the key assumptions and estimates which went into the analysis.[27] The greater the sensitivity of the outcome to variations in some particular parameter, the more important it is that care is taken with the estimation and interpretation of that parameter.

If we conceive of health care technology in terms of drugs, devices, medical and surgical techniques and the organisational procedures and support systems used in the delivery of health care, it is clear that CBA could then, in theory, be applied to all those aspects of the health sector. However, given the problems associated with quantifying and then attaching monetary values to changes in health, other approaches to the evaluation of investments in health care have been developed by economists.

A range of economic evaluation tools have been developed which can illuminate the costs and benefits of alternative investments in health care technologies. These methods include what is known as 'cost-minimisation analysis' and 'cost-effectiveness analysis'. Health economists have endeavoured to modify these tools of economic analysis specifically to the evaluation of health care technologies and they have also created an additional tool, which is known as 'cost-utility analysis'. These different kinds of tools will now be considered.

Economic methods for evaluating health care technologies

Cost-benefit analysis

Within a health care context, cost-benefit analysis can be used to compare the estimates of the costs and benefits of a single health care technology or a range of different health care technologies. With regard to the cost-benefit analysis of health care technologies, these can be broken into different examples of cost:

- direct costs (eg hospital staff and equipment costs);
- indirect costs (eg production losses from a patient having to take time off work);
- intangible costs (eg anxiety of undergoing a surgical operation).

Quantifying and then assigning monetary values to health changes usually involves surveys of the public's willingness to pay for technologies to provide improved health care, or their willingness to pay to avoid the risk of premature death or spending time in an impoverished state of health. Although some authors have identified many philosophical and technical problems associated with the quantification of health benefits, others have argued that the problems of attaching monetary values to health outcomes are no greater than those which arise when people try to attach monetary values to environmental changes, in environmental health impact assessments.[28] There is, however, an extensive literature which argues that such problems are in turn very substantial, or even insurmountable.[29,30,31,32,33]

Unlike cost-benefit analysis, which is carried out from a societal perspective, the following three methods of economic evaluation usually complement an NHS perspective. These methods address questions of technical rather than allocative efficiency in the production of health care technologies.

Cost-minimisation analysis

Cost-minimisation analysis is used where the health outcomes of two or more health care technologies are known to be identical, and so a simple comparison of costs indicates which health care technology is more financially efficient. This method of economic evaluation is infrequently used as there are few circumstances where the health outcomes of different health care technologies can be assumed, with certainty, to be identical. It has been used, however, to compare brand and generic drugs.

Cost-effectiveness analysis

Cost-effectiveness analysis compares the costs and consequences of two or more health care technologies in terms of cost per appropriate unit of effectiveness. For example, where two drugs for the reduction of blood cholesterol are being compared, their effectiveness might be measured in terms of the cost per specified reduction in blood cholesterol level achieved. Such ratios can be used to inform decisions about the relative cost-effectiveness of treating patients with the same condition, in this example, patients with hypercholesterolaemia. Other ratios which might be used to determine the relative cost-effectiveness of health care interventions are: cost per case detected, cost per death averted and cost per admission avoided.

Cost-effectiveness analysis can also be used to compare patients with different conditions. However, ratios used in this way tend to be based on crude measures of effectiveness, for example, cost per life year gained. Counting additional life years gained does not take account of the *quality* of life in which these years are spent, and so decisions may be based on partial and incomplete information.[34]

Cost-utility analysis

Utility is a term used by economists to measure well-being. Cost-utility analysis in the health care context is used to compare the costs of different health care technologies with the health related well-being which they provide. This method attempts to address the inadequacy of simply using additional years of life gained to describe the effectiveness of a health care technology.

The Quality Adjusted Life Year (QALY) is probably the best known of a range of indices (eg Healthy Year Equivalents,[35] Disability Adjusted Life Years[36]), which aim to combine the changes in life expectancy and health related quality of life resulting from a health care technology. It is an example of a type of cost-utility analysis. In the calculation of the QALY gain from a health care technology, additional years of life are weighted by a value between 0 and 1 to reflect the quality of life in which they are spent. A variety of methods have been developed by health economists to arrive at these weightings. The most common approach is where samples of the population are asked to state to what extent they prefer a range of different states of health described to them. The methods used include: visual analogue methods, time trade-off methods and standard gamble methods.[37]

Calculating the estimated health gains from a health care technology can be carried out very simply. If treatment A increases a patient's life expectancy, on average, by 5 years and these 5 years are spent in perfect health (1.0), then the QALY gains from treatment A are calculated by multiplying the number of additional years of life gained by a weight which appropriately reflects the quality of life in which these additional years are spent. In this example 5 QALYs are generated (5 x1.0 = 5). If treatment B increases a patient's life expectancy by 5 years and these 5 years are spent in less than perfect health (eg 0.6) then the QALY gains from treatment B are 3 QALYs (5 x 0.6 = 3).

It is becoming increasingly common to use league tables to compare the cost-effectiveness and cost-utility of health care technologies. The idea is that resources should be invested in health care technologies which produce QALYs at low cost.[38] However, in the field of health economics there is much controversy over their usefulness as there are many methodological questions and problems which must be addressed before meaningful comparisons can be made.

Relative QALY gains from two health care technologies are represented diagrammatically in Figure 6,[40] which has been adapted from a paper by Williams, who estimated QALY gains from coronary artery bypass grafting.[39] The diagram represents a model that can be applied to any health care technology.

- The x-axis shows life expectancy in years.
- The y-axis shows health related quality of life on a 0 to 1 scale where 0 represents, the worse possible health state and 1 represents the best possible health state.
- Schedule A represents expected average period of survival as a function of health-related quality of life with a particular treatment 'X'.
- Schedule B represents the same relationship, but without treatment 'X' though with usual care.
- Schedule C shows mortality with treatment 'X' (ie those patients for whom treatment 'X' is fatal).
- The shaded area indicates the average health gain in terms of quality adjusted life years for the application of treatment 'X'.

Currently, diagrammatic representations of health gains have only been produced within a medical context for health care technologies. If, however, investments in sectors other than the health-care sector can be shown to have direct and measurable effects on health, and if QALY gains could be calculated, such analyses and diagrams could possibly be incorporated into environmental health impact assessments.

Application of the methods of health economic evaluation to health impact assessment

Within a culture of evidence-based medicine and cost-effective purchasing in the NHS internal market, the methods of economic evaluation described above are already being widely used.[41,42] It has been argued that restricting economic evaluation to health care technologies within the health sector may be generating an incomplete picture of what constitutes an efficient use of resources for the promotion of health.[43] In other words, preventing ill-health by improving environmental conditions may sometimes be more

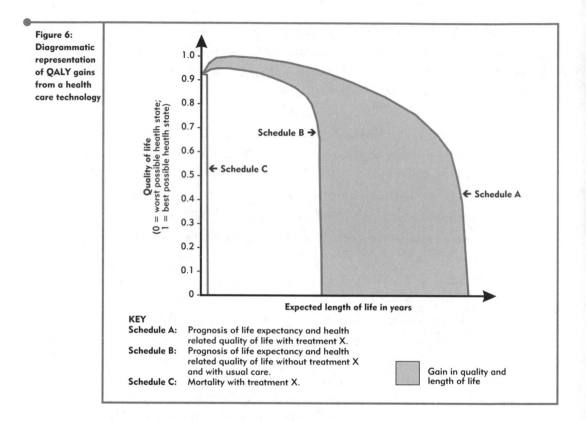

Figure 6: Diagrammatic representation of QALY gains from a health care technology

KEY

Schedule A: Prognosis of life expectancy and health related quality of life with treatment X.

Schedule B: Prognosis of life expectancy and health related quality of life without treatment X and with usual care.

Schedule C: Mortality with treatment X.

Gain in quality and length of life

beneficial in both health and financial terms than meeting the costs of treating those made unhealthy by their environment.

Department of Health's guide to policy appraisal and health

In 1992 the government published its *Health of the Nation*[44] strategy in which goals for improving the health of the population of England and Wales by the year 2000 were established. This strategy represented a shift away from policies for remedial medical services towards policies based on targets for reducing levels of illness with the introduction of 'Healthy Settings'. The concept of 'Healthy Settings' recognise that health is dependent upon the individual's physical and social environments. The change implies that health can best be improved by supporting work in multidisciplinary and multisectoral partnerships with a commitment to increasing community involvement in decision making.

More recent government documents, for example *Fit for the Future*,[45] *Variations in Health*[46] and *Our Healthier Nation*,[47] have taken a similar view. They highlight the fact that the Department of Health and the National Health Service can only provide one part of a public sector health policy. *Our Healthier Nation*[48] outlines four key areas where environmental factors are considered to have an impact on public health — air quality, housing, water quality and social environment. It recognises that 'connected problems require joined up solutions'; however, the use of categories such as 'The Social and Economic Case', 'Environmental' and 'Lifestyle' can be seen as purely arbitrary from a health impact assessment view. For example, under 'Social and Economic Factors' they use the following example: 'if the street outside your home is busy with traffic, or there are drug dealers in the park, then it's safer to keep the kids in front of the TV than let them out to play....' This might equally be placed under 'Environmental' factors, since a housing estate might suffer from a high level of deprivation, but equally mitigation measures could have been undertaken if a HIA had been carried out to adequately assess impacts to human health at the inception of the housing development or road building scheme.

In order to support policy makers in other departments, the Department of Health has published guidelines on how health effects can be incorporated into broader policy appraisal. The document *Policy Appraisal and Health*[49] advocates the use of many of the methods of economic evaluation developed in the field of health economics to identify, measure and value the health effects of non-health sector programmes, policies and projects. In order to do this, the document has set out a simple five-step plan for policy makers to follow. They are encouraged to identify any health impacts, assess their magnitude, value them in monetary terms where this is helpful, identify the main sources of uncertainty in the analysis, and present the results clearly for decision makers. Overall, the *Policy Appraisal and Health* document supports, where possible, the use of a cost-benefit approach in policy appraisal.

The steps for guiding policy makers are modelled on some of those normally followed in the course of health impact assessments. However, by endorsing attempts to quantify health impacts, and to ascribe monetary values to those impacts, the document goes one step further than most health impact assessments. It also suggests that HIAs can and should be conducted using techniques some of which are untried, untested, contentious and contested. The guidance which the document provides begs a complex set of conceptual and methodological issues, without detailed comment or justification. In particular, the following areas of concern need to be addressed:

- The issue of establishing causality. The document glosses over the problem that, if non-health sectoral investments influence health, but do not have health as their primary goal, it will be very difficult to establish causal relationships between investments and changes in health.

- The use of QALYs to quantify the health effects of policies.

- Attaching monetary values to QALYs; and quantifying the health effect of policies. Given the many philosophical and technical criticisms of QALYs,[50,51] such an endorsement of the use of QALYs may be regarded as somewhat premature. To date, QALYs have been associated with monetary units only in so far as a few researchers have tried calculating how much it costs to generate a QALY. Attaching monetary values to QALYs is an approach which has yet to be tried and tested and has not yet been validated in the health economics literature. Nor has it been judged acceptable by the broader academic community or the general public.

Estimates of QALYs, and changes in QALYs, may well deserve to be counted as what mathematicians call 'ordinal' because the figures can be presented as a set of integral numbers, but that does not mean that QALY figures are what mathematicians refer to as 'homogeneous', 'uniform' or 'metric'. QALY figures would be homogeneous if, for example, a 2-point difference had precisely the same meaning in all contexts and at all points on a QALY scale. A difference between a QALY figure of, for example, 3 and 5 is not, however, necessarily the same as that between 63 and 65. Some people would contend that adding two years of good healthy living to the life of a 3-year-old child is more precious than providing a 63-year-old with two more decent years. Similarly, QALY figures are not necessarily 'metric' in the sense that if a treatment extends the expected comfortable life of recipients by one year when the alternative without treatment is abrupt death, this may be more valuable than using the same resources on treatments which extend comfortable life expectancy from 50 to 51 years. Furthermore, if one treatment provides a QALY gain of 3, a second provides a gain of 6 and the third of 9, we cannot necessarily say that the difference between the first and second treatments is exactly the same as that between the second and the third treatments, nor that the difference between the first and the third treatments is precisely twice that of either of the first two treatments.

Given resource constraints within the public sector, the document *Policy Appraisal and Health*[52] appears to favour an evaluative approach to the appraisal of both health and non-health sector policies based upon economic cost-benefit analyses. The problem is, however, that it pretends that all aspects of health impacts can be evaluated using one single consolidating monetary measure. The proposal that policy judgements over a broad range of areas should be informed by an assessment of their potential impacts on public health is entirely welcome, but it is understandable that many commentators have reservations about the intelligibility and acceptability of representing all costs and all benefits in monetary terms.

The perspective and analytical framework which environmental health impact assessment can provide is highly appropriate as a guide to policy makers, both within and outside the health care sector. Trying to go beyond the mere identification of health impacts, and trying also to estimate their extent and magnitude, can provide information which would enrich many decision-making processes. Estimating the economic consequences, and seeking to quantify both adverse and beneficial health impacts of policy proposals by combining the techniques of health impact assessment and of health economics will be immensely helpful. It remains to be seen, however, how far it will be possible and acceptable to represent all the relevant variables in monetary terms.

Health impact assessment and health economics: scope for interdisciplinary collaboration

Health Impact assessment (HIA), as a component in environmental impact assessments, focuses on the identification of health hazards and the estimation of the likely impact on health of some proposed development. The focus of HIA is therefore most commonly on the negative influences on health and how policies might be adjusted to effectively minimise and manage risks to health.[53] This can be contrasted with the focus of economic evaluations in the health care sector which commonly focuses on attempts to measure the positive impact on health of health care technologies on life expectancy and/or health-related quality of life.

The extent to which quantitative measures of health outcomes may in the future contribute to health impact assessments will depend on several factors. Firstly, it will depend on whether attention is given by health economists to negative health impacts in health impact assessments. To date, there has been no research into the inversion of the Quality Adjusted Life Year and therefore the application of QALYs in the field of health impact assessment has yet to be investigated. Further research must be carried out in order to establish many of the causal relationships between non-health sectoral policies and consequent health impacts.

Health economists perhaps lack a sufficiently broad perspective for evaluation policies which affect the health of the population, as they tend to focus only on evaluating the allocative efficiency of remedial health care technologies in medical practice. It is common knowledge, however, that the receipt of treatment is only one factor in determining public health.[54] Health economists could perhaps benefit from greater knowledge of the scoping and screening techniques used in the identification of health impacts in the context of HIAs. Some collaboration is already taking place between health economists and the practitioners of other disciplines. For example, research is being undertaken at the Centre for Urban and Regional Research at the University of Sussex into the costs and benefits of good quality housing when cross sectoral savings and the better protection of housing asset values are taken into account.[55] A case study of 10 municipal tower blocks in Sheffield demonstrated how investment in energy efficiency can lead to reduced poverty, better quality of life and might improve health status.[56]

It has recently been recognised that unless the focus of health economics is broadened, and methods of economic evaluation are used to evaluate the health gains from investments outside the health-care sector, then health economists will be increasingly restricted to contributing to policies for health care, while excluded from all other areas of policy.[57,58] It is also evident that those professionally involved in health impact assessment would benefit from becoming more familiar with the tools of economic evaluation as they are used by health economists, to see how they can be used to evaluate the health impacts of other areas of policy. Interdisciplinary collaboration should enhance the research agendas of health economics and health impact assessment.

6

Human health and the environment: policies for the next millennium

Introduction

It is a measure of the extent of professional and public concern about environmental health that in 1988 the British Medical Association Board of Science and Education was asked to establish working parties to study the possible effects of pesticides and chemicals on human health in the UK, the potential health risk from hazardous waste, and environmental and occupational risks of the health care industry. The pesticides and chemicals report[1] emphasised two important findings: firstly the incompleteness of existing knowledge concerning the effects of chemical exposure on human health; and secondly the lack of a central government strategy, in particular concerning the use of pesticide chemicals in the UK.

The BMA therefore welcomed the joint announcement by the Agriculture, Environment and Health Departments that an action plan developed by the Pesticides Forum,[2] an independent advisory group, to reduce the impact of pesticides on the environment and human health will be introduced in the UK. The plan aims to promote responsible use of pesticides, the effective transfer of improved technologies and techniques to farmers, and to encourage new training initiatives. The Health and Safety Executive plans to carry out a long-term study of pesticide users' health, which aims to fill the "significant gaps in our knowledge concerning both acute and (especially) chronic health effects of pesticide use".[3]

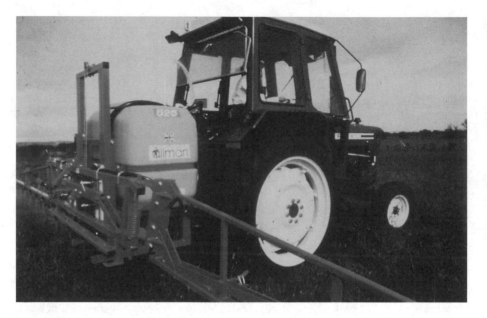

More information is needed about the effects of pesticide exposure on health

The existence of hazardous wastes has always been a problem, particularly since the start of the industrial revolution. From the beginnings of organised society, wastes and dangerous by-products have been created which have to be disposed of safely. The 1950s saw a rapid growth of the chemical industry and a corresponding increase in the number and volume of toxic chemicals in the environment. By the mid-1980s, over 6 million chemical substances had been created, of which about 95,000 are in commercial use today.[4] Disposing of all forms of waste has been a constant challenge for society with relatively few choices for routes of disposal available: essentially landfill, incineration and disposal at sea. In the 1991 report *Hazardous Waste and Human Health*,[5] the BMA indicated future directions reflecting the salutary remark of Immanuel Kant (1724-1804) that: "it is often necessary to take a decision on the basis of knowledge sufficient for action, but insufficient to satisfy the intellect".

The UK has often been criticised for its tardiness in adopting strategies of waste reduction and the reclamation of wastes. The US Environmental Protection Agency and the Office of Technology Assessment found that the UK lagged behind its European counterparts in France, Germany, Sweden, Norway, Denmark, the Netherlands and Austria in the minimisation of wastes.[6,7]

The BMA highlighted the need for more research into the nature of the health risks of exposure to hazardous waste. Even though some data may be difficult to obtain, it is possible to maintain good practice on the basis of a sensible estimation of the risk involved. This means finding out as much as possible about the physical or chemical properties of the wastes produced, the nature of exposure to them, and the probable outcome of exposure in terms of health. Doctors have an important part to play in providing early warning where a health problem is suspected, and may also be involved, together with other professionals, in the collection of information and research. Careful monitoring and research based on clinical observation is crucial in assessing and managing risks. The final step is to devise a practical way of controlling and managing risk.[8]

The implementation of the European Directive on Waste Packaging (94/62/EC) was expected to have a major impact on packaging companies, retailers and consumers in the UK and it should contribute significantly towards reducing the amount of material sent to landfill — with ultimate savings for industry, local authorities and others charged with paying a landfill tax since 1 October 1996. The EU Directive seeks to improve the management of packaging and packaging waste to protect the environment, but it is not clear whether these new regulations will also lead to improved protection for human health.

Air pollution arising from the disposal of wastes, and also from the burning of fossil fuels, has become an important issue. Objections to incineration are largely based on the poor performance and objectionable emissions from many old or poorly maintained incinerators and fears that dioxins and other toxic substances may be released when some plastics and other substances are incinerated. One difficulty faced by governments and

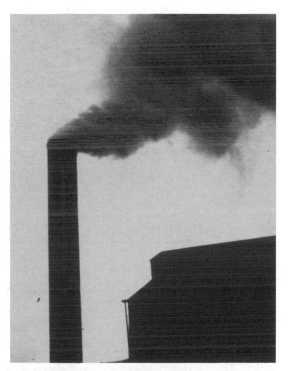

The health impact of air pollution arising from the burning of hazardous waste has become an important issue

enforcement agencies arises from the fact that we still have insufficient data on individual chemicals and their possible human toxicity. For example, there are some studies on the links between dioxins and cancer but much of the data available concerns animal studies and the true biological effects in humans are difficult to interpret.[9] Such direct knowledge as we have of the possible effects on the general population relies to a large degree on cases of accidental exposure to relatively high levels of dioxins as occurred following the Seveso incident in Italy 20 years ago. In that particular incident, however, the lack of a population-based cancer registry which might have provided reliable baseline data caused major problems for epidemiologists, and this may have led to under-estimation of the numbers of resultant cancer cases. Many such reports involve relatively small numbers of people, but even in cases like the explosion at the pesticide manufacturing plant at Bhopal in India, very little information is usually available on the levels of exposure which the victims received.[10] As a consequence, studies of accidental emissions can rarely provide definitive information or conclusions.

The medical profession has a major role to play in exploring risks to human health so that hazards can be controlled or eliminated. Recommendations published by the BMA on the environment have called for all doctors to take part in "managing the environment in the interests of public health".[11] The BMA has long argued that the health care sector should put its own house in order and published a report on the environmental and occupational risks associated with the health care industry.[12] The recommendations are likely to have influenced the NHS Executive in producing health service guidelines on occupational health services for NHS staff[13] and on clinical waste management.[14]

Environmental health

Health in its widest sense incorporates all aspects of human welfare and means much more than simply the absence of disease. The UK Government[15] defines 'Environmental Health' as "...those aspects of human health, including quality of life, that are determined by physical, biological, social and psycho-social factors in the environment". The government has also referred in the most general terms to the "theory and practice of assessing, correcting, controlling and preventing those factors in the environment that can potentially affect adversely the health of present and future generations".[16] This constitutes an acknowledgement of the multi-dimensional nature of health and of the importance of ensuring equity between generations. The promotion of good health therefore requires not only public policies which support health, but also the creation of supportive environments in which "living and working conditions are safe, stimulating, satisfying and enjoyable".[17] Healthy environments and healthy populations are therefore interdependent. Ensuring that environmental degradation will not occur and that public health will not be adversely affected by planning decisions, however, requires more than the publication of general pragmatic remarks, it also involves the active maintenance, and where appropriate promotion, of health through improved social amenities and living and working environments.

The BMA is encouraged that environmental health issues now form a regular feature of the Chief Medical Officer's Annual Reports *On the State of the Public Health*. The 1994 report[18] commented: "This report is not simply a document of record, but must also try to interpret and to explain changes in those factors that are known to influence and to determine health, and should identify areas where improvements could be made". The CMO Annual Report for the year 1995,[19] identified several key environmental health issues of concern including:

- asthma and air pollution and the health effects of airborne particles;
- safety initiatives in relation to food, pesticides and genetically modified plants;
- the long term effects of organophosphate chemicals on those carrying out sheep dipping;
- potential health effects of radioactive particles found near a nuclear establishment;
- health effects of relatively low levels of chemicals in the environment, and
- actions to be taken after major chemical accidents.

That greater emphasis is being given to environmental health issues is shown by the increased coverage within the CMO's Annual Report, for the year 1996.[20] The section on environmental health and food safety highlighted issues relating to:

- air pollution and health;
- accidents involving radioactivity;

- health effects of chemicals in the environment;
- the preparation of an environmental health action plan;
- food poisoning and developments in food surveillance and food hazard management;
- safety of genetically modified (GM) foods such as oilseed rape, maize and Vitamin B_2 derived from GM *bacillus subtilis*;
- the health effects of phthalate and other chemical contamination of infant foodstuffs; and
- pesticides, organophosphate sheep dips and the human safety aspects of veterinary medicines and materials in animal feedstuffs.

Environmental impact assessments

This report has examined the development of the environmental impact assessment process, and the rationale and procedures which should be followed when an EIA is undertaken. Some of the failings of the current procedures have been outlined and explored. The most significant of these is that although EIAs should take a holistic approach, including human health, the focus is primarily confined to the physical, chemical and biological environment, while human health is only referred to, if at all, indirectly.

Despite these limitations, environmental impact assessments could provide a valuable means for ensuring that a consideration of the impact on public health is included within the decision-making criteria of developers, planners, officials, councillors and ministers. Not only have EIAs been required by legislation in many parts of the world, but the methodology of EIAs should include an integrated analysis of complex, cross-sectoral issues which affect all components of the environment, including human health. Considerable progress has already been made in some countries in integrating formal procedures for health impact assessments within EIA processes. We have considered in detail some of the ways in which positive and negative aspects of health, and the expertise of health specialists, can be more fully integrated into the EIA processes.

There is increasing pressure for EIAs to be applied to the highest levels of the policy-making and planning processes, such as to ministerial policies, national, regional and sectoral plans and programmes through what is coming to be called 'strategic environmental assessment' (SEA). SEA can provide a framework within which wider issues of natural resource conservation and sustainability can be addressed.[21,22] An EU Directive on SEA is under consideration,[23] but further drafting is likely to be required before the scope of the draft Directive contains adequate provision for dealing with the implications of policy, plans and programmes for human health, safety and risk.[24]

The issue of when an environmental hazard becomes a health issue is difficult to define. The range of consequences for human health may cover an individual whose quality of life has been compromised by the development of a new road in a rural area, to the dispersal of a toxic agent which can lead to acute and/or chronic illness amongst some members of the general public.

The complexity of many environmental hazards demands cross-sectoral approaches to safeguard health. One of the main difficulties in incorporating human health more directly in environmental impact assessments, however, has been a lack of an adequate dialogue between those in the health care professions and those concerned with environmental regulation.

There are now many organisations with an interest in health and environmental issues and it is not easy to identify precisely where responsibilities for environmental health lie. There is no single government department which is responsible for the whole environmental health function, and there is no clear framework for addressing many of the

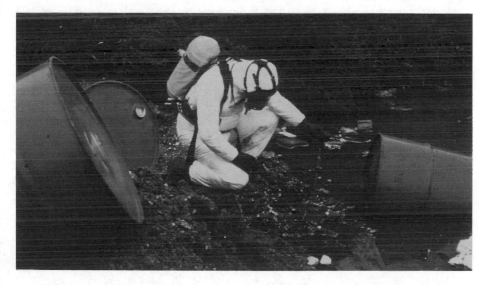

Accidental spillage and dispersal of toxic agents may lead to acute and/or chronic ill health

more complex environmental health issues, particularly those of a cumulative or trans-boundary nature. However, the BMA welcomes the appointment of a Minister for Public Health and the restructured Department of the Environment, Transport and the Regions and the improved liaison between the Agriculture, Environment and Health Departments. In the past there has been a tendency for governments to try to reduce environmental hazards by focusing on reducing specific emissions in a piecemeal fashion, without addressing the overall implications. An integrated approach to environmental and health impact assessment can better take account of interactions between different pollutants, cumulative effects of low-level releases, levels of exposure for people in the receiving environment and their relative vulnerabilities to adverse effects. Both the Environment Agency and the recently proposed Food Standards Agency will have a crucial role in further protecting public health.

The way ahead

The ability to recognise, characterise, estimate and ameliorate adverse environmental health impacts is likely to be amongst some of the most pressing challenges facing national governments, industries and the public into the next century. Governments should be aiming to implement revised and enhanced procedures, rather than maintaining the status quo. Further investments in research and development are required to improve monitoring technology and early warning diagnostics. Similarly, planners, geographers and ecologists should try to refine their methods for environmental monitoring. Both community groups and public officials should try to ensure that there is effective public participation in the planning and development policy-making processes. Particular attention will need to be paid to monitoring the impacts which could be attributed to projects once development has been permitted. This should help establish whether mitigation measures are being implemented and how effective they turn out to be.[25]

There will continue to be an important role for environmental and occupational health professionals and for the medical profession, particularly public health and occupational physicians. Environmental and occupational diseases encompass a wide range of human illness and are amongst the most important causes of disability and death in modern society. The full nature and extent of the health burden resulting from occupational and environmental exposure remains to be elucidated, but our understanding would benefit from improved links between toxicology and epidemiology. This will enable our knowledge about the possible effects, particularly of low level exposures to asbestos, benzene, organic dusts, radon, solvents, lead, and to pesticides and other agents, to expand. Building upon those developments, health economists will have a valuable contribution to make in quantifying health impacts.

Medical practitioners, however, may be inadequately prepared to respond to the growing need for clinical services that address the real and perceived problems of environmentally related illness. Physicians are one of the most trusted, but possibly less well informed, sources of information about the risks of chemical exposure.[26,27] This gap between trust and knowledge must be narrowed and although this is now being addressed by some undergraduate courses, further changes in medical education are needed both at the undergraduate and postgraduate level, particularly for those in the fields of occupational, environmental medicine and risk assessment. Public health physicians have an important role which could be enhanced by further training, including specialisation in environmental issues. These topics were addressed in the 1995 Annual Report of the Chief Medical Officer who commented:

"Infections and environmental hazards, procedures, investigations or drug treatments do carry risks. Some people may not wish to take any risks in spite of the possibility of real benefit. Others will take a chance, even when the benefit is likely to be very low. The problem for decision makers is not when the evidence is clear, but when it is weak or incomplete. In such instances there is a need for openness and sharing of information, and the establishment of trust between those who make policy and the public at large". The British Medical Association concurs firmly with this view and will continue to work closely with the Department of Health, and other appropriate government departments, in ensuring that priority is given to this issue.

Looking forward to the 21st century, the 1992 United Nations Conference on Environment and Development established 'Agenda 21', which sets out what nations need to do to achieve sustainable development in the medium term (see Appendix 5). This has provided a basis for placing environmental considerations high on the public policy agenda. There has not yet, however, been a sufficiently widespread recognition of the importance of the relationship between public health and the state of, and changes to, the environment.

Recommendations

National policies for environmental and health impact assessment

1   **The UK Town and Country Planning Regulations, and the guidance issued by the Department of the Environment, Transport and the Regions (DETR), and by the Highways Agency, should be amended to include an explicit and formal requirement for an assessment of the potential impacts on human health of all proposed developments requiring an environmental impact assessment (EIA) for planning purposes. No EIA should be deemed to be adequate unless it shows evidence that possible implications for occupational and public health have been properly addressed. March 1999 should be set as the target for the introduction of this requirement, in order to coincide with the deadline for implementation of EIA Directive 97/11/EC within the UK.** There has been a failure explicitly to include human health as a component of all EIAs and this has created problems with the promotion of health impact assessment (HIA), which ought to play a more prominent role in safeguarding health in the development planning process both at a national, regional and local level. The present situation, whereby HIAs are treated separately, if at all, rather than as an integral part of EIAs is unsustainable. HIA should be considered as an integral component of the EIA process, rather than as a separate and parallel activity, because of the importance of developing an integrated approach to health and the environment.

2   **The Department of the Environment, Transport and the Regions and the Department of Health must ensure that strategic environmental assessment (SEA) including specific provision for the assessment of impacts on human health is carried out for all public policies, programmes and plans which have implications for the environment and human health.** For example, environmental policies such as those relating to transport or air quality, and social and economic policies, such as VAT on domestic fuel, will fall under this provision. A draft EC Directive on SEA[28] is currently being considered which, if adopted,

should enable the consideration of impacts on the environment, health and social well-being to be achieved in a more holistic way. The draft SEA Directive presently focuses on assessment of the cumulative impacts of numerous individual projects which are undertaken as part of a larger scale plan or programme. However, it also provides an opportunity to introduce mechanisms to assess the health and environmental impact of all future public policy.

3   **The Government's new strategy for the nation's health, *Our Healthier Nation*,[29] should address explicitly the influences of environmental conditions on human health, together with an overall comprehensive strategy for impact assessment.** The document commits the Government to undertake health impact assessment of relevant key policies, but gives no criteria for deciding relevance, nor does it propose a strategy for implementation.

4   **The Environment Agency must adopt a fully integrated approach in all its activities which acknowledges the relationship between the health of the environment and the health of the population. To do this, the Agency should appoint a medical officer at each regional level with specific responsibilities for the human health aspects of environmental quality.** The majority of the Agency's functions with regard to the protection of the environment ultimately have an impact upon health and it is often the impact upon human health that determines the setting of standards and actions required with regard to the environment. The Agency should contribute to the development of an integrated environmental and health impact assessment methodology, and provide guidance on environmental health monitoring and assessment techniques. The Agency's work in assessing the impacts of pollution, and carrying out environmental assessments of new and existing chemicals, should provide valuable data for health and environmental impact assessments. The Chemical Release Inventory could also provide an effective monitoring, surveillance and analytical tool for those with an interest in environmental and public health.

5   **The Department of the Environment, Transport and the Regions and the Department of Health must ensure that the development of an integrated**

environmental health impact assessment process is included as part of the UK's National Environmental Health Action Plan (NEHAP). NEHAP should be rewritten to include specific mechanisms by which environmental health issues can be addressed as part of the planning authorisation process and at the strategic level of policy appraisal.

6 **Communication between professionals in the health care sector and those concerned with environmental protection and regulation needs to be improved. The Minister for Public Health, Chief Medical Officer and other senior officials, such as the Chief Scientific Officer, and the Environment Minister (as Chairman of the 'Green Ministers' Group') should participate in initiatives to ensure improved communication and consultation between all the agencies concerned with human health and the environment; this could include establishing a formal consultative committee.** Such a committee must maintain close links with the Sustainable Development Unit which has been introduced to support all Departments in assessing the potential environmental impacts of new Government policy proposals. One important new initiative to strengthen communication in this area would be for the Annual Report from the Chief Medical Officer to include a specific section on the conduct and continuing methodological development of health impact assessments.

Research

7 **A systematic and comprehensive programme of research is required to develop the methodologies with which HIA can be conducted. A consortium should be established to fund, commission and direct that research.** The membership of that consortium should include the Department of the Environment, Transport and the Regions, the Department of Health, the Natural Environment Research Council, the Medical Research Council, the Biotechnology and Biological Sciences Research Council, the Economic and Social Research Council, the Environment Agency and the Royal Commission on Environmental Pollution.

8   **The present situation whereby no groups of researchers in the UK are funded specifically to undertake research into health impact assessment must be urgently addressed.** The programme of work should be conducted by research teams comprising a diverse range of specialists including health economists and those from the natural, medical and social sciences.

9   **A structure for strategic and project-level health impact assessment methodologies should be developed. This should begin at the strategic policy level. The structured approach developed at this level should then be retained in developing project-level methodologies, taking account of the practical levels of information available at the different levels.**

10   **A systematic review of the health hazards associated with a series of programmes, policies and projects in each sector should be carried out to assess their health risks. A comprehensive checklist should then be produced to guide developers and planning authorities.** Hazards both directly and indirectly associated with the development should be included in the checklist. The importance of each hazard should be determined according to its frequency and severity. The checklist should also include sociological factors and perceived hazards for which there is little or no evidence, but high public concern. Such a checklist if used as part of the EIA process would enhance the predictive power of further health impact assessments.

11   **There should be an ongoing case study analysis of current and future HIAs in order to identify good practice. Information gained will assist the continuing development of HIA methodology, help to define concepts, and provide models for future health impact assessments to follow.** Such studies could usefully include a systematic review of UK planning applications to determine the extent to which human health is being addressed within the planning process, but also to clarify the relationship between planning procedures, inquiries and the conduct of HIAs within the EIA process. This work would help to define the boundaries within which a health impact assessment should be carried out.

12   **There is an urgent need for much more epidemiological surveillance both of occupationally exposed groups and of the general population.** The case for more systematic epidemiology starting from, but extending beyond, occupational settings has repeatedly been emphasised by the BMA. Occupational settings have the methodological advantage that people are often exposed in the course of their employment to relatively high concentrations of potentially hazardous materials and activities, and for relatively long periods of time. Consequently, a thorough scrutiny of occupational settings can provide early warning signs of hazards to which the broader population may in due course also be exposed. Occupational and general epidemiology will therefore be important both for the conduct of HIAs and for research into ways of improving the methodologies of HIAs by providing baseline data sets against which the impact of proposed changes may be assessed.   Laboratory and bench research is also required, with particular consideration given to:

● the development of new markers for monitoring and surveillance of health impact;

● improved estimates of exposure both for individuals and populations;

● better methods for extrapolating risk to populations, together with the ecological basis for risk assessment;

● exposure to, and effects of, mixtures of chemicals.

The design and conduct of EIAs and HIAs

13   **The screening criteria used for determining when a project requires an EIA, as set out in the UK Town and Country Planning Regulations, and contained within the guidance issued by the Department of the Environment, Transport and the Regions, and by the Highways Agency, should be revised so that potentially significant impacts on human health are included more explicitly.** Only limited guidance is available on different project types and locations and, in practice, there has been considerable inconsistency in determining the eligibility of Schedule 2 projects for EIA. The lack of inclusion of health hazards and risks within the project screening process can contribute to failure of the planning

authorities to require the assessment of health impacts for a proposal. Explicit reference to the need to screen projects for potential risks to human health would mean that the discretion currently exercised by local planning authorities will become more carefully circumscribed.

14   **'Scoping' should become a legal, mandatory requirement for all UK EIAs and HIAs.** Scoping procedures are used to determine the range of issues which should be addressed in the EIA and to identify those issues which are potentially adversely affected by the development and should therefore be studied in detail. Scoping also benefits developers, because careful scoping reduces unnecessary expenditures on research into issues which are not particularly relevant to decision-making, thus enabling resources to be allocated most effectively.

15   **Health should always be one of the issues to be included within the scoping stage of an EIA. If health is to be adequately addressed, the potential health hazards of a project must be systematically and comprehensively identified at the scoping stage and a detailed list drawn up so that these may be adequately investigated.** There is currently no comprehensive check list of the human health hazards that could be consulted during the scoping process. However, the BMA has proposed five working categories for health hazard identification: communicable disease; non-communicable disease; inappropriate nutrition; injury and mental disorder. Other categories may be added, such as special hazards to the developing foetus and children, or categories for indirect impacts on health such as those arising from social impacts. Information about health hazards is at present incomplete but current sources include reviews of similar projects elsewhere, opinions of specialists, the public and other stakeholders, published literature reviews identifying known health hazards within each sector, maps and local and national health data. In addition, lessons can be learned from bad scoping examples, such as EIAs of reservoir projects which have, for example, focused in a limited way on water-borne diseases without taking account of other potential health impacts that can be associated with such developments.

16   **The draft terms of reference for the consultant who will carry out the environmental and health impact assessments should be made available for public comment as part of the early consultation process.** This may also include review by the developer, relevant competent authority, other relevant agencies and authorities, affected parties and interest groups.

17   **The terms of reference for conducting an EIA should always specifically indicate how the health risks which may be associated with the project are to be identified and how the consultant should assess these health risks.** In addition, the terms of reference should require the consultant to include any other health hazards which may be discovered during the study. The provision of adequate terms of reference is important, since consultants will often only report what is required by their terms of reference. Statutory provision and guidelines on the terms of reference are required to ensure that the following components are addressed by the consultant in preparing the environmental impact statement:

- Identifying potential health hazards according to categories of communicable disease, non-communicable disease, inappropriate nutrition, injury and mental disorders;
- Identifying potentially vulnerable communities and describing why they are vulnerable;
- Identifying the environmental factors responsible for exposure of vulnerable communities to hazards;
- Describing the capacities and capabilities of the many agencies responsible for protecting health in relation to the project and identifying their limitations;
- Reaching a conclusion based on the above regarding the change in health risk reasonably attributable to the project ranked at least as a trend of increasing/decreasing or no change;
- Recommending health safeguards and mitigation measures in sufficient detail to be given serious consideration, including outline costs.

18   **The Department of Health and the Department of the Environment, Transport and the Regions (DETR) and the local authorities should ensure that adequate consultation takes place as early as possible and continues throughout the EIA and HIA process to ensure that all important information is fully considered and all relevant interests in, and aspects of, the development are properly explored.** Consultation at an early stage in the project cycle allows preliminary plans to be modified, if necessary, to take account of findings from the consultation process. Lack of early consultation and discussion is a major limitation to effective health and environmental impact assessment. The DETR recommends that developers consult with the competent authority and statutory consultees before preparing the environmental impact statement, but this does not always take place in practice. The new EC Directive[30] places greater emphasis on consultation throughout the EIA process. In particular, information gathered as part of the EIA process must be made available to the public within a reasonable time in order to give the public concerned the opportunity to express an opinion before the development consent is granted. Furthermore, when a decision to grant or refuse development consent has been taken, the competent authority or authorities must inform the public, and make available to the public specific information regarding the content of the decision, including a description of the main measures to avoid, reduce and offset any major adverse effects of the development.

19   **Local authorities should work jointly with health authorities to appoint statutory consultees with appropriate expertise in health-related issues to participate in environmental and health impact assessments. Within five years, all Health Authorities should appoint a consultant in public health medicine with expertise in environmental issues who would have a specific role as statutory consultee in the environmental and health impact assessment processes. Occupational health physicians and consultants in communicable disease control should also act as statutory consultees in relation to risks to occupational health and communicable disease transmission. Regular and effective consultation must also take place with environmental health officers**

and others eg, local directors of public health, to ensure effective integration of HIA. Greater resources may be needed to enable environmental health officers to contribute to the environment and health impact assessment process. Under the present system, local planning officials are expected to consult with the Health and Safety Executive in circumstances where a proposed development involves "manufacture, processing and storage of hazardous substances."[31] The Environment Agency is a statutory consultee in circumstances where a proposal involves "works specified in Schedule 1 to the Health and Safety (Emissions to the Atmosphere) Regulations 1983".[32] However, such consultations may not always take place. In addition, there is no statutory consultee for developments involving other health-related issues, thus increasing the risk of their omission from the EIA process.

20   **Health and social welfare specialists should be represented on specially convened panels which are set up to appraise environmental impact statements (EIS), once they have been prepared and submitted by the consultant to the competent authority. Currently, the local Directors of Public Health, public health physicians and environmental health officers may have a role to play in appraising the EIS.** Consideration should be given to developing a specialty within public health related to environmental issues, which would strengthen links between toxicologists, epidemiologists and planning authorities with regard to the appraisal and subsequent management of health risks. Occupational health physicians may also be able to provide a valuable source of expertise on appraisal panels to address the health risks from industrial developments. This would facilitate the integration of environmental and health input at the appraisal stage.

21   **Developers should make specific provision for mitigation measures to avoid, remedy or reduce any significant adverse impacts associated with the project, especially those with potentially significant impacts on environmental quality, occupational or public health. The subsequent performance of those measures should then be monitored by the developer, and this monitoring reviewed as part of a follow-on assessment, after an appropriate period, eg 5 years.** This

would determine the effectiveness of the mitigation measures, and provide information for future projects.

22   **Local authorities should use planning conditions to ensure that adequate mitigation measures are undertaken by the developer, and should specify that developers earmark specific resources to ensure that concurrent and post-project environmental monitoring and epidemiological surveillance take place. The results of such monitoring and surveillance should be published.** At present there is no formal requirement for monitoring of the impacts attributable to the project, or the subsequent effectiveness of mitigation measures, once development consent has been granted. Such monitoring and surveillance would enable the local authority to establish whether the proposed mitigation measures had been effective, and identify any previously unforeseen risks or benefits associated with the project.

23   **The Department of the Environment, Transport and the Regions in collaboration with the Department of Health should review the practice and conduct of EIA and HIA, together with the outcome of any mitigation measures and 5-yearly follow-on assessments in order to establish and disseminate guidelines on best practice.** The information gained from such a review should be used to improve the design, methodology and conduct of future environmental and health impact assessments and to circulate guidance on the effectiveness of mitigation measures based on past experience. In 1997 the DETR published the results of a study which showed that the treatment of mitigation within a sample of 100 EIAs was mostly only fair, with a third of the statements rating poor or worse.[33]

Decision-making

24   **Wherever possible, decisions regarding the environment and health should be evidence-based.** However, given the lack of adequate empirical data, and the need to await further research results, the BMA believes that in conducting EIAs and HIAs, and in interpreting the results, a precautionary approach should always

be taken. Local authority planning officials should exercise their discretion to request further studies and more data, but in conditions where ignorance and uncertainty prevail they should err on the side of caution and safety rather than expose the environment and public health to indeterminate risks and hazards.

25   **When an EIA or HIA is completed, the subsequent report should always include a summary in non-technical language to enable members of the general public to gain an appreciation of the issues involved and the conclusions reached.** This should improve the accessibility of information for the public.

Policies for the corporate sector

26   **The Department of Trade and Industry, the Department of the Environment, Transport and the Regions, as well as trade organisations, should consider how national and international quality assurance standards such as ISO 9000, ISO 14000, and BS7750 can be applied more formally to the impact assessment process in the UK.** Such standards provide methods for assessing the capability of project proponents to protect human health as part of their proposed development plans. Commercial organisations can contribute to the improvement of environmental conditions and public health, to some extent, by requiring that they, and their suppliers of both goods and services including environmental consultants, should act in accordance with national and international quality assurance standards such as ISO 9000, ISO 14000, and BS7750. All businesses, including small and medium size firms, can help protect the environment and human health through waste reduction and recycling, solvent management and the cost effective use of raw materials.

27   **Businesses should be provided with continuing and extended support to enable them to minimise the environmental and health impacts of their activities.** They may well benefit from the kind of help that is provided, for example, by the Environmental Technology Best Practice Programme which offers advice on environmental management tools, such as monitoring, and life-cycle assessment.

Education and training

28   **Universities and training providers should ensure that the design and conduct of EIAs and HIAs are comprehensively addressed in the relevant educational courses.** The results of the research which we are proposing should serve both to improve the design and conduct of EIAs and HIAs, but also contribute to improving the education and training of the relevant professionals in health care, environmental health officers and planning officials.

29   **It is recommended that the syllabus for undergraduate medical education in the UK should include a significant element of education in toxicology and environmental health, and that the theme of public health medicine and occupational medicine should figure prominently in the undergraduate curriculum of medical students.** These changes are already underway, but need to be developed, particularly to encompass health promotion and illness prevention, and the assessment and targeting of population needs as well as awareness of environmental and social factors in disease, in accordance with the recommendations of the General Medical Council report, *Tomorrow's Doctors*.[34] This theme within the syllabus should also include an awareness of the methodology for, and interpretation of, health impact assessments.

30   **Postgraduate education and training courses on environmental and health impact assessments should be provided for a broad range of professionals.** Such courses should be available to all doctors, but especially public health physicians and local directors of public health who may be required to act as expert statutory consultees for health-related issues to be addressed by a health impact assessment. Public health physicians, in particular, should have a familiarity with the essential steps in the assessment of risk, and they should receive training, including continuing education in all specialties related to environmental toxicology and environmental health. Other relevant groups include local authority planning officers, those employed by the regulatory and enforcement agencies, such as the HSE, environmental health officers, occupational health physicians and public health officers who are likely to be

required to give expert advice on health impact assessment to development consultants. Intensive short courses (eg for 1-2 weeks) should be available, which could be taken by a wide range of professionals and trainees as part of continuing professional development programmes. The results of the research into environmental and health impact assessment should contribute to improving such education and training programmes.

Appendix 1

The evolution of public health legislation

Public Health management involves organised attempts to understand the determinants of good and poor health and to improve the level of health, in part by reducing inequalities within populations. The sustained and explicit management of public health had its origins in England and came as a direct response to recognition of the wider environmental influences on the health of the people. Many of these arose from the rapid expansion of urban populations associated with the process of industrialisation in Britain in the nineteenth century. Crowded living conditions, poor housing, poor water quality, dangerous work environments and air pollution all had adverse effects on health, and there was widespread malnutrition and infectious disease.

The effects of certain occupations on the health of the workforce have been observed over many years. Yet the idea that centralised action was necessary to control some of the dangers associated with the workplace did not gain acceptance until the early nineteenth century, and even then there was considerable opposition to the aims of the reformers. The public health movement, which arose at this time, concerned itself not only with sanitary reform, clean water, effective sewage disposal and proper housing — but also with dangers encountered at work. However, despite Sir Robert Peel's factory legislation, the Health and Morals of Apprentices Act (1802), which concerned hours of work, and standards of cleanliness and education, injuries and deaths caused by factory machinery continued to be common. In 1844 The Factories Act laid down regulations for fencing and protecting machinery and appointed certifying surgeons, to investigate accidents at work.

In 1842 The British Parliament commissioned Edwin Chadwick, an engineer, to review the 'sanitary conditions of the labouring poor'. His report stimulated far-reaching social reforms in sanitation, personal hygiene and housing design. The first Public Health Act followed in 1848, enshrining "the notion of State responsibility for the public's health" for the first time.[1] The provision of public health services, exemplified by the appointment of

Medical Officers of Health in local authorities throughout the UK, was established by the middle of the nineteenth century.

Specific health-directed interventions took place within a broader matrix of social progress and economic development that contributed to their effectiveness in improving public health. An obvious indicator of the improving public health was the steady decline in death rates (by about three-quarters between 1840 and 1940);[2,3] that impressive fall in death rates from a number of infectious diseases came before the introduction of effective anti-microbial therapy and immunisation. McKeown concluded that limitation of family size, increases in food supplies and a healthier physical environment contributed more to improvements in health in England and Wales than specific preventative and therapeutic measures, though these still played a part.

Some of the key stages in the evolution of legislation with a role in regulating impacts on human health are listed in Table 9.

Table 9: Some key international and UK developments in environmental health management and assessment

Date	Development
1802	Health and Morals of Apprentices Act
1844	Factories Act
1848	Public Health Act
1863	Alkali Act (to control emissions of noxious gases from alkali works)
1872	Public Health Act: appointment of sanitary inspectors (forerunners of environmental health officers)
1875	Sale of Foods and Drugs Act
1936	Public Health Act
1945, 1948	Water Acts
1956, 1968	Clean Air Acts
1971	Town and Country Planning Act
1972	Town and Country Planning (Scotland) Act and Planning (Northern Ireland) Order 1972. Stockholm Conference on the Human Environment
1973	Water Act

1974	Health and Safety at Work etc Act, Control of Pollution Act
1984	European *Health for All* strategy set nine targets directly concerned with aspects of environmental health. Control of Industrial Major Accidents and Hazards Regulations
1987	World Commission on Environment and Development
1989	First European Conference on Environment and Health, Frankfurt-am-Main, Federal Republic of Germany: adoption of the European Charter on Environment and Health
1990	Environmental Protection Act
1992	United Nations Conference on Environment and Development, Rio de Janeiro. Rio Conference endorsed Agenda 21, an action plan for the twenty-first century which acknowledged that to achieve sustainable development, major changes in approach are required if health impairment due to environmental degradation is to be arrested and future adverse environmental impacts on health prevented.
1993	World Health Assembly endorses a global strategy for health and the environment in response to Agenda 21 which accepts that health impacts are an important part of the immense environmental problems facing Europe.
1994	World Conference on the Environment. Second European Conference on the Environment and Health, Helsinki — at which the WHO European Centre for Environment and Health resolved to assess all aspects of environmental health in the countries of the Region, based on available national data — report published in 1995 as *Concern for Europe's Tomorrow*.[4]
1995	Environment Act
1996	Publication of UK National Environmental Health Action Plan
1997	Appointment of Minister for Public Health in the UK. White Paper on *The New NHS*,[5] proposes a strategic role for health authorities, in partnership with local authorities to identify and take action on social, environmental and economic issues which impact on the health of local people. This is to include "evaluating the health impact of local plans and developments".
1998	White Paper on *Our Healthier Nation* aimed to improve the health of the population as a whole by increasing the length of people's lives and the number of years people spend free from illness and to improve the health of the worst off in society and to narrow the "health gap". Four priority areas were identified: heart disease and stroke, accidents, cancer and mental health. To achieve these objectives the strategy commits the government to carry out health impact assessment of relevant key policies so that when they are being developed and implemented, the consequences of those policies on health are addressed.[6]

Appendix 2

Duties of a doctor in occupational medicine

The British Medical Association Occupational Health Committee report, *The Occupational Physician*,[7] lists the duties of a doctor in occupational medicine as follows:

The effects of health state on capacity for work

- counselling and giving advice to all employees on health as related to their capacity for specific and general work;
- initial placement. Special consideration of the handicapped prospective employee is required, as is liaison with help agencies, to ensure that the working environment is suitable;
- interviewing, and examining where indicated, after prolonged or serious illness or accident. Doctors may consider recommending part-time or restricted work, rehabilitation, redeployment or retirement on health grounds;
- giving advice to management on health promotion and general health screening, and making arrangements for this to be carried out where appropriate.

The effects of work on health

- giving advice to management and committees within the organisation on all health aspects of the working environment, the medical implications of health and safety legislation, and the significance of hazards to health at work, for instance those identified under the Control of Substances Hazardous to Health (COSHH) regulations;

- being aware of toxic hazards and the COSHH assessments that have been made. There may be a necessity for periodic medical examination under COSHH and other statutory regulations;

- undertaking regular but informal visits to all workplaces, including offices and kitchens, in order to keep workplace knowledge up to date, and establish contact with employees of all grades; working contacts with personnel, safety and employee representatives are valuable;

- having responsibility for organisation, in conjunction with management, of first aid and emergency services within the workplace; this will include arranging for the immediate treatment of medical and surgical emergencies and should be made in conjunction with the nearest hospital accident and emergency department, which should be aware of any toxic chemical hazards which exist in the workplace. (The Health and Safety at Work etc Act 1974 and its regulations, codes of practice and guidance notes are appropriate and contact with the Health and Safety Executive's local Employment Medical Advisory Service should be made);

- supervision of the hygiene and safety of facilities such as canteens, kitchens and laboratories;

- undertaking health education and health promotion work with employers on health, fitness and hygiene issues.

Appendix 3

Recommended target maximum levels for pollutants listed in the *UK National Air Quality Strategy*

The United Kingdom National Air Quality Strategy[8] covers those pollutants which are known to have adverse effects on human health in sufficiently high concentrations and occur in many parts of the UK. Many of the pollutants can also damage natural environments and buildings. The list of pollutants covered by the strategy is not necessarily exhaustive and may be extended in the light of further research as this strategy is reviewed and rolled forward.

The Pollutants

BENZENE: Studies of benzene, at concentrations much greater than those found in ambient air in the UK today, suggest that it can cause leukaemia, a type of cancer. The risk is related to overall lifetime exposures. At ambient concentrations, benzene does not have short-term or acute effects. The Expert Panel on Air Quality Standards (EPAQS) recommended air quality standard, of 5 parts per billion (ppb) as a running annual average, represents a level at which the risk to health is exceedingly small, and unlikely to be detectable by any practicable means. This standard should be reduced to the lower level of 1ppb running annual average and set as a target in the future.[9]

1,3-BUTADIENE: Again there is evidence that 1,3-butadiene can cause lymphomas and leukaemia, both of which are types of cancer. EPAQS has recommended a standard of 1ppb as a running and annual average. As with benzene, this represents a level at which the risks to human health are judged to be exceedingly small.

CARBON MONOXIDE: At today's typical ambient levels the effect is slight, but carbon monoxide can have effects on mental activity, and may also worsen existing problems which affect the delivery of oxygen to the heart or brain. EPAQS recommends an air quality standard of 10ppm as an 8 hour running average. The standard is lower than the level at which effects are observed, allowing a safety margin, and corresponds to the most stringent of the WHO recommended guidelines.

LEAD: Levels of lead in blood arise from lead in air, water and food. Lead can affect many different parts of the body including the production of blood, the nervous system and mental functioning. Children are most susceptible. EPAQS has not, as yet, recommended guidelines for lead emissions. In the interim the Government proposes to adopt the WHO guideline of $0.5\mu g/m^3$-$1.0\mu g/m^3$ as an annual mean and has set the standard as $0.5\mu g/m^3$ annual average. The WHO target is based on assuring that at least 98% of the exposed population have blood lead levels below 10 g/dl. At such levels any effects are very subtle.

NITROGEN DIOXIDE: High exposures can affect the way that the lungs and airways function. There remains concern that it may also increase the risk of respiratory problems and reactivity to natural allergens. EPAQS recommends an hourly average of 150ppb for Nitrogen Dioxide (21ppb or less, when expressed as an annual mean). There is insufficient evidence for a longer term standard.[10] The two air quality standards for Nitrogen Dioxide recommended by WHO are: a maximum hourly mean of 104.6 ppb and a maximum annual mean of 20ppb. The hourly standard is based on the lowest levels at which acute effects have been observed, with a margin for uncertainty about the effect of repeated high exposures and the effect on severe asthmatics. The annual mean, recommended by WHO, is a precautionary measure as some studies have suggested that prolonged exposures may have chronic effects.

OZONE: Ozone is an irritant at the levels often found in the UK. It can inflame airways, lead to sore eyes and throats and increase sensitivity to allergens such as pollen. People who suffer from asthma do not appear to be significantly more sensitive to ozone than other people. Current evidence does not suggest chronic effects at typical UK levels. The EPAQS recommended an air quality standard of 50ppb as an 8 hour running average. The standard is lower than the level at which effects have been detected experimentally in healthy individuals, and the WHO recommended guideline of 60ppb, to include a margin of safety for individuals most at risk.

PARTICLES: At the levels found in the UK, there is no evidence of effects on people in good health. However, it is likely that extremely small particles (below 10 microns PM_{10}) from any origin can worsen heart and breathing problems in sensitive groups. Effects range from days of restricted activity to premature mortality. EPAQS recommended an air quality standard of $50\mu g/m^3$ as a 24 hour running average, and that annual average levels of particles should be progressively reduced.

SULPHUR DIOXIDE: At the levels sometimes found in the UK, sulphur dioxide is an irritant, which can cause a reflex cough, a feeling of chest tightness and narrowing of the airways. The effect is more likely to occur in people suffering from asthma and chronic lung disease. Evidence on the longer-term effects, such as the possibility that exposure to sulphur dioxide actually causes lung disease, is inconclusive. EPAQS recommended an air quality standard of 100 ppb as a 15 minute mean value.

Appendix 4

Life-cycle assessment

Life-cycle assessment (LCA) is a tool used to indicate the potential environmental burdens that the life-cycle of any product or service places on the 'global' environment. Systems analysis is utilised to consider both the inputs to a system, ie materials and energy, and the outputs of that system, ie emissions to land, air and water, within a defined boundary. One of the advantages of using this type of analysis is that 'problem-shifting' within a system's boundary cannot occur as the burdens are calculated from 'cradle to grave'. LCA is a young discipline and further methodological development is needed, together with more data, before it can realise its full potential

     There are four stages to LCA:

1   the definition of study objectives, the functional unit of study and the boundaries of the system under study, known as goal definition and scoping;

2   the identification and quantification of all material and energy flows into and out of the system, known as inventory analysis;

3   the interpretation of the material and energy flows as potential effects on the environment, known as life-cycle impact assessment;

4   the identification of points in the system under study where it is possible to make environmental improvements.

     A life-cycle inventory (LCI) involves the first two stages of LCA as outlined above, ie goal definition and inventory analysis. The outcome of performing an LCI is an inventory of the 'global' environmental burdens associated with the product or service under study.

     The techniques of LCI are now fairly well established and have been used with increasing frequency by many manufacturers to optimise the environmental performance of individual products, including packaging, over the product's life-cycle from the extraction of raw materials through to manufacture, distribution and use and final disposal. However, it is also possible to apply the techniques of LCI to the improvement of the environmental burdens associated with certain systems of management, eg waste management. In this type of application, LCI becomes a tool not only for the optimisation of a system of management, but also one that can be used to evaluate various policy options for either local or national government and/or other institutions and companies.

The use of, and the methodologies for, the final two stages of LCA, ie life-cycle impact assessment and improvement analysis — are the subjects of considerable debate at present, which have yet to be resolved. It should be noted that the results provided by an LCI are not accurate measures of environmental impacts *per se* because:

- generic data are used to calculate the potential burdens;
- the resulting inventory data are not specific to either points in time or points in space, ie actual sites or locations where emissions occur.

Packaging

Packaging is a popular subject of study using one or more of the various forms of environmental assessment.[11] It has been suggested that packaging may often be regarded as an 'environmental problem' because everybody has direct knowledge or experience of packaging; as such, it is easier for people to relate to it, especially when compared with other environmental problems which have 'supra-local' effects, such as acid rain or global warming.[12] However, packaging is also a product that performs an important function in society: it enables the safe distribution of various goods from the point of manufacture to the point of end-use, such that the item protected by that packaging retains its integrity up until the point of use. For the purposes of this report, packaging on products from the healthcare sector will form the focus for an illustration of the environmental impact of packaging, and the ways in which those impacts can be reduced.

The primary functions of packaging for food and beverages are:

- to contain the product until use for transport, distribution and storage purposes;
- to maintain product quality;

- to maintain product safety.

These functions act to:
- protect the public health;
- reduce wastage, both at the point of end-use and as a result of damage to goods during transit or storage;
- reduce the cost of food and other products.[13]

The primary functions of packaging for medical devices are the same as those for food and beverage packaging, with one important additional function affecting numerous devices:

- to maintain and indicate product sterility.

With the need to reduce to a minimum the problem of cross-infection as a result of providing healthcare, and within the context of a medical system based on the practice of universal precautions, this function is of paramount importance. However, the method of sterilisation will often determine the materials used in and the design of the packaging because medical devices are sterilised within the primary packaging to ensure the quality of sterility.

The volume impact of medical packaging waste in landfill sites in the USA has been estimated as less than 1%.[14] Although it represents only a small fraction of waste when compared with other types of packaging waste, it is still possible to use some of the tools for the assessment of environmental impact in order to manage and thereby minimise the impacts as identified (see example below).

Example: The use of 'eco-design' to reduce the impact of medical device packaging

One of the most pressing issues being faced by the healthcare sector today is the generation and subsequent management of solid waste. As the stringency of environmental and associated legislation increases, and the costs of any form of waste disposal increase, the managers of healthcare facilities are beginning to explore the options not only for integrated solid waste management, but also for waste minimisation and waste avoidance. However, some of the possibilities for waste minimisation and waste avoidance require the collaboration and coordination of several members of the healthcare supply chain. As such, the managers of healthcare facilities will have to work with industry in order to identify opportunities for the reduction of environmental impact of components of the solid waste stream. One such component is packaging.

In the USA, legislation developed by the Coalition of Northeastern Governors (CONEG) recognises source reduction as a major component of any system set up for the management of solid waste. The Environmental Protection Agency (EPA) of the USA defines source reduction as:

"the design and manufacture of products and packaging with minimum
toxic content, minimum volume of material, and/or a longer useful life".

Source reduction also appears at the apex of an hierarchy of options for integrated solid waste management outlined by the EPA, as follows:

- source reduction;
- recycling;
- selective landfilling.

All of these options present the packaging engineer with opportunities to be explored when designing the packaging. If source reduction is decided upon as an appropriate option for certain types of packaging, the techniques that can be applied include:

- down-gauging of film to reduce the overall volume of the package;
- reducing the size of the package;
- eliminating one of the wraps in double-wrap packages;
- selecting materials that give a higher yield from a lower basis weight.

If recycling is identified as a suitable option for the recovery of medical packaging waste (as long as it is not contaminated with infectious or other hazardous wastes, eg with chemotherapeutic or radioactive materials), most medical packaging could be entered into a recycling waste stream. Apart from latex-saturated/reinforced or clay-coated papers, most papers in medical packaging are ideal for recycling.

As can be seen, there are opportunities to use 'eco-design' to minimise the environmental impact of medical device packaging, but it requires close liaison and cooperation between end-users, manufacturers and raw materials suppliers within the entire healthcare supply chain.

Appendix 5

Environmental impact assessment: the global scene •

EIA systems can be found in many countries. However, the nature of the systems vary, due to differences in the particular country's resource base, institutional framework for environmental protection and the development plans concerned. In spite of these differences, knowledge of the role of international organisations, and an overview of EIA systems in other countries, can be helpful in placing the UK EIA procedures into context. It should be noted that EIA is an emerging methodology throughout the world, which needs support both from international organisations as well as governments of individual countries. With this in mind, we should not waste the opportunity to learn from other countries, which can provide valuable comparative experience which may be useful for the further development of EIA systems, not only within the UK, but throughout the world.

Sadler[15] refers to the steady process of 'internationalisation and institutionalisation' which has characterised EIA since its inception. The scope of the EIA process, ie the range of actions and types of impact covered by legislation, and the methods used to assess and evaluate impact, vary in detail between countries, but the general principles are the same. Detailed accounts of the origins and evolution of EIA can be found in books by Wood[16] and Vanclay and Bronstein.[17] There is also a useful summary in the report by Sadler[18] which presents the findings of an international study of the effectiveness of environmental assessment carried out under the auspices of the International Association for Impact Assessment (IAIA) and the Canadian Environmental Assessment Agency. The United States of America was the first country to enact legislation requiring assessment of potential environmental impacts by proponents of development actions. The National Environmental Policy Act (NEPA) was passed in 1970 and has provided a template for similar legislation elsewhere in the world. Key stages in the worldwide adoption of EIA legislation are listed below.

Table 10: Key stages in the worldwide adoption of EIA legislation

Date	Key stages
1970	United States National Environment Policy Act (NEPA)
1973-4	Canada, Australia and New Zealand follow the NEPA example.
1970s	Further industrial and developing countries introduce formal EIA requirements, including France (1976) and the Philippines (1977). Others use EIA informally or experimentally (eg the Netherlands, from 1978) or adopt elements of the EIA process, such as impact statements as part of development applications for planning permission (eg Ireland).
1985	European Union Directive on EIA establishes minimum provisions for compliance by member states.
1988	EU Directive implemented in the UK.
1989	EIAs become a standard requirement for all World Bank financed investment projects. (The primary responsibility for compliance with World Bank requirements lies with borrowing countries. As a result of these and similar requirements by other development banks and donors, EIA has since come into wide use in developing countries.)
1990s	Increasing emphasis on regulation of global problems, eg the Epsoo Convention (1991) requires consideration of trans-boundary effects. EIA is identified as an implementing mechanism for UN conventions on climate change and biological diversity. Legislation for strategic environmental assessment (SEA) is established by an increasing number of countries (eg Australia). Long-standing EIA regimes are overhauled (eg in Canada and New Zealand). Increasing legislation for EIA in 'developing' and 'transitional' countries.
1991	A series of draft European Directives on strategic environmental assessment (SEA) appear, which cover policies, programmes and plans.
1992	The Earth Summit results in a supra-structure of international law and policy that promotes the use of EIA in signatory countries.
1997	European Directive on EIA is revised to tighten and extend many of the provisions of the original directive, particularly with regard to screening to determine whether or not projects should be subject to an EIA.
	Revised draft of the European Directive on SEA from which the coverage of policies has been removed. The Directive now only covers the assessment of the effects of certain plans and programmes on the environment.

Several converging factors led to the introduction of EIA in the US in 1970.[19,20] These included:

- a tradition of rational planning;
- new levels of public concern about the environment;
- increasing scale and wider repercussions of major development schemes;
- failure of existing project appraisal and review procedures to account for evident impacts on ecosystems and human communities.

Recognition of the fact that economic development activity could have consequences for the wellbeing of human individuals and communities was therefore one of the key catalysts for the formal introduction of EIAs. Consideration of the potential impacts on people has remained embodied in the principles of EIAs throughout the world, but very little attention has been paid to the integrated assessment of impacts on ecosystems and human communities.

The following section focuses on the kinds of EIAs which are required by European and UK legislation and it emphasises the lack of explicit attention given to the assessment of impacts on human health.

Agenda 21

In June 1992, the United Nations Conference on Environment and Development (UNCED) was held in Rio de Janeiro. The outputs of the conference included a declaration of principles on environment and development and an agenda for change during the 21st century, referred to as Agenda 21. The principles state:

"Nations shall enact effective environmental laws and develop national law regarding liability for the victims of pollution and other environmental damage. Where they have authority, nations shall assess the environmental impact of proposed activities that are likely to have a significant adverse impact."

Agenda 21 acknowledges the dependence of human health on a healthy environment. It requires all countries to have programmes to identify environmental health hazards and to reduce the risks.

Agenda 21 has been used as a priority setting tool for the policies of many international agencies. In the context of urban pollution, there are references to environmental health impact assessment as a tool to help determine pollution control, prevention and abatement measures; this tool should be used for the planning and development of new industries and energy facilities and should include health risk analysis and strategies to improve occupational health and safety. In the context of health research, there are references to the need for national strategies for the integrated environmental control of communicable diseases and the need to identify the unique problems of vulnerable groups.[21,22]

Local Agenda 21

Agenda 21 singles out local government as having a special role in sustainable development. Two thirds of the actions in Agenda 21 require the active involvement of local authorities. Chapter 28 of Agenda 21 calls on them to initiate the Local Agenda 21 by developing local policies for sustainable development in partnership with other sectors and to implement them by 1996. In the UK the Local Agenda 21 initiative is managed by the local authority associations in England and Wales, Combined Organisation of Scottish Local Authorities and Association of Local Authorities in Northern Ireland who have joined in setting up a Local Agenda 21 Steering Group representing industry, trades unions, the voluntary sectors, women's organisations and higher education as well as local government. The overall process is being coordinated by the Local Government Management Board.

It is intended that Local Agenda 21 will be a continuing process rather than a single event, document or activity. The Local Government Management Board (LGMB) survey in 1996 confirmed that 90.6% local authorities are undertaking a Local Agenda 21 process with their communities. A further study is being undertaken to produce in the first year 40 studies of Local Agenda 21 cases. The project will be overseen by a steering group and comprises voluntary sector organisations, LGMB and the Local Government Associations. The object of the study is to present examples of good/interesting practice and pool expertise and experience in this area.

World Health Organisation

The WHO has long been aware of the implications of health impact assessment. In 1986, the 39th World Health Assembly called on all member states to:

- identify and develop health objectives as an integral part of sectoral policies for agriculture, the environment, education, water, housing and other health-related sectors, and to include health impact analyses in all feasibility studies of all health-related programmes and projects;

- include in their health-for-all strategy specific equity-oriented targets expressed in terms of improved health among disadvantaged groups such as women, the rural poor, the inhabitants of urban slums, and people engaged in hazardous occupations;

- encourage and support action-oriented multidisciplinary research focusing on socioeconomic and environmental determinants of health in order to identify cost-effective intersectoral actions for improving the health status of disadvantaged groups;

- strengthen the capacity within the health sector at national and local levels to identify vulnerable groups, assess health hazards as experienced by different groups, monitor health conditions within the population, and assist other health-related sectors to formulate and evaluate intersectoral actions for health.[23]

The European Office of the World Health Organisation has been actively engaged in the promotion of health impact assessment under the guidance of Dr Eric Giroult since the 1980s. The principle concern has been chemical safety and pollution associated with industrial processes.[24] One activity has been the active promotion of courses in EIA with a health component, in the University of Aberdeen.

In 1995, the WHO European office published an extensive text *Concern for Europe's tomorrow: health and the environment* which aims to provide a balanced and objective overview of the principal environmental issues of present or potential concern for health in the WHO European Region. The report acknowledges that in terms of environmental protection, the anticipation and avoidance of potential harm not only benefit human health and well-being, but are almost always more cost-effective than later environmental clean-up and treatment of disease. Such preventive action involves many different areas of government, including agriculture, energy production, housing, industry, land use and urban planning, and transport. At present, the frequent absence of a multisectoral approach to environmental health management, and the lack of effective coordination of action, results in socioeconomic development having impacts on the environment that adversely affect the health and well-being of the population. The report attempts to facilitate the reversal of these practices by presenting an overall picture of the effects on health of environmental conditions throughout the European Region. The report makes a number of key recommendations including the need to reduce the uncertainties in risk assessment, better information on population exposure and better understanding of the links between environment and health. This would be facilitated by countries sharing information systems, to provide an objective basis for decision making across the Region.[25]

Concern about the communicable diseases associated with water resource development in Africa and elsewhere led to the creation, in 1981, of the joint World Health Organisation/Food and Agriculture Organisation/United Nations Environmental Programme/United Nations Centre for Human Settlement (WHO/FAO/UNEP/UNCHS) Panel of Experts on Environmental Management for Vector Control (PEEM), with a secretariat in WHO headquarters, Geneva. For many years PEEM has been ably managed by Mr Robert Bos and it consists of a network of about 40 members worldwide. Promotion of health impact assessment is a growing part of its activities. These have included publication of a series of relevant manuals including Guidelines for Forecasting the Vector-Borne Disease Implications of Water Resources Development.[26] More recently, a training course has been developed in collaboration with the Danish Bilharziasis Laboratory and the Liverpool Health Impact Programme entitled "Health opportunities in water resource development".[27,28] The course has run in a number of developing countries.

In 1990, WHO collaborated with the World Bank in a published review of the impact of development policies on health.[29] A number of other more general texts are also relevant.[30] In order to underline the linkage between environment, health and development, WHO has indicated a preference for the term environmental health impact assessment (EHIA).

In the Eastern Mediterranean Region, the Centre for Environmental Health Activities of WHO which is based in Amman, Jordan, has collaborated with the Liverpool Health Impact Programme to run a series of advocacy workshops at regional and national level to promote EHIA. Environmental laws, Environmental Protection Agencies and EIA procedures are at an early stage in many countries of the region. Attention has been focused on incorporation of health in the EIA framework.

In the Western Pacific Region, the Environmental Health criteria (EHC) Office of WHO which is based in Kuala Lumpur, Malaysia, has run a series of regional and national workshops on EHIA. Some of these have also been in collaboration with the Liverpool Health Impact Programme. In this region the focus has been on the risk assessment of industrial processes. Case study materials are being developed for use in future training courses.

Overseas Development Administration

The Environmental Division of the Overseas Development Administration have published an environmental manual to guide the assessment of development projects.[31] This guide includes a brief reference to human health. From 1990 to 1995, the Health and Population Division of ODA supported the Liverpool Health Impact Programme (HIP) at Liverpool School of Tropical Medicine. The remit of this programme was advocacy of health impact assessment, technical assistance, training courses, research and publication. One output of the programme was a book entitled *The health impact assessment of development projects*.[32]

Asian Development Bank

The Environmental Division of the Asian Development Bank, based in Manilla, Philippines, has published a number of guidelines on aspects of impact assessment. These include environmental and social impact and environmental risk assessment as well as guidelines for the health impact assessment of development projects.[33] To date, there has been no published review of the way in which these guidelines have been used to aid development project decisions.

World Bank

The World Bank, based in Washington, USA, has a series of operational directives backed up by an Environmental Sourcebook that relate to the impacts of its projects. There is no specific Bank policy on health and safety; these are subsumed under a general policy that projects should improve quality of life. The Sourcebooks summarise many of the problems associated with human health that must be addressed if health and safety are to be fully integrated in EIA. These books emphasise the cross-cutting nature of health and safety and the weakness of the health sector in many countries. A Sourcebook Update has been prepared that takes the process of integration of environmental and health impact assessment one step closer by proposing that public health and safety concerns should be addressed more systematically in screening, scoping, terms of reference preparation and report appraisal procedures.[34] Many existing World Bank project environmental assessments include some references to health. A recent paper has reviewed infrastructure projects in Sub-Saharan Africa and concluded that there were considerable opportunities for using them to improve human health.[35] Other World Bank publications of relevance include the review of health impacts in developing country cities, cited earlier.[36]

Commonwealth Secretariat

At the 1992 meeting of Commonwealth Ministers of Health, concern was expressed about the health impacts of development and a programme of work was initiated. The main objective of the programme has been the production of training materials for use in Commonwealth countries that could be used by non-health specialists and local communities. Later work was directed towards identifying the skills needed for environmental health impact assessment at each stage of the EIA process, identifying the training needs for the promotion of those skills and planning the content of core training materials.[37,38]

International Association for Impact Assessment

The International Association for Impact Assessment (IAIA) was founded in the USA in 1980 and promotes the integration of impact assessments of all kinds. It has a European regional chapter, members in 95 countries (at time of writing) and holds annual meetings around the world. There has been some discussion of health impact assessment in the association's journal. In 1995, the IAIA published an edited book that included chapters on social, demographic, ecological and risk assessment, in addition to a chapter on the health impact assessment of development projects that contains numerous additional references to those reviewed here.[39,40,41,42] The IAIA also hosts several unmoderated Internet discussions of impact assessment, including one focused on the European region.

Developing countries

The main differences between health impact assessment in economically developed and developing countries are levels of uncertainty associated with:

- lower availability of data;
- differences in the complexity and extent of infrastructure and management systems.

For example, an irrigation project in a remote rural district of an African country may be planned in an area with no road, no functioning health care, no health statistics, no domestic water supply, no latrines and little or no cash economy. The lack of data increases the uncertainties associated with the analysis, but the lack of infrastructure increases the certainty that impacts can be attributed to the project. Subsistence agriculturists with few capital reserves and no state support are more obviously vulnerable than a British urban community. A change in communicable disease risk from 40% to 50% in the village is more compelling than a change in non-communicable disease risk from 0.004% to 0.005% in a British city. The absolute number of people affected may be higher in the city than in the rural village, but the marginal costs of the rural project to the local health sector will be very high and significant compared with the low marginal costs to the NHS and social services.

Because of the simpler infrastructure and the larger percentage change in the overall risk, the rural community provides a test-bed for the evolution of ideas. In addition, the dose-response relationship for communicable diseases is far more complex than for non-communicable diseases and requires a more holistic method of analysis. This may explain why health impact assessment of development projects has received greater attention. However, it is still not a routine component of development or a widely appreciated concept among development agencies.

Australia

In 1992 a national framework document for health impact assessment in environmental impact assessment was published in Australia as part of the National Better Health Program.[43] This concluded that an environmental health impact assessment process was essential and that existing procedures, resources, knowledge and skills were inadequate. The main focus was on non-communicable diseases associated with pollution. It described the administrative context, the processes required and the resource needs. It also established principles, tasks and responsibilities for public health authorities, assessing authorities, project proponents, the public and government. It paid particular attention to risk analysis and risk communication, defining risk as a socially constructed phenomenon rather than a technical and objective property of a hazard.

New Zealand

In 1995 the New Zealand Public Health Commission published a guide to health impact assessment.[44] This provides a framework for those concerned with resource management issues which have a potential to impact on the health of communities and individuals. It seeks to establish principles and processes for identifying health hazards arising from proposed resource management policies, plans or consent applications; to identify roles and responsibilities; and to identify sources of information which will assist in the assessment of health effects. The steps in the HIA process were summarised as follows:

Preliminary analysis

Screening: Does the proposal need an HIA? Is there the potential for cumulative effects from successive proposals?

Scoping: What issues must be addressed in the HIA?

Profiling: What is the current health status of the affected population and the quality of the local environment?

Risk analysis

Risk assessment: What are the risks and/or benefits? Who will be affected, how and to what extent?

Risk communication: Has there been adequate consultation on the risks? Have public concerns been taken into account?

Risk management: How can the risks be avoided or reduced? What are the options (including costs and benefits) for treating the risks? Are contingency/emergency plans adequate? How can differing perceptions of risk be mediated? Can future health risks be predicted?

Implementation

Decision making: Is there adequate information for decision making? Is there a conflict to be resolved? How will conditions be enforced and by whom? How and by whom will effects be monitored? How will post-project management be resourced?

Monitoring: Is the project complying with its conditions? Are the conditions achieving the desired outcomes?

Auditing: How well is the HIA process achieving its aims?

This is a well presented guide that contains much that is relevant to the UK setting. The guide refers to communicable diseases, non-communicable diseases and injury but the main emphasis is the risk assessment of pollutants based on dose-response relationships, accurate exposure measurement and analysis of uncertainty. This is elaborated in a second guide.[45] The overall procedure advocated is similar to our own but there is less emphasis on describing why communities are vulnerable and no analysis of the existing capacity and capability of health protection agencies. To some extent this latter point is dealt with in the discussion on HIA auditing.

Canada

In Canada a series of workshops were held in 1995 to discuss the role of health professionals in EIA, known in Canada as EA.[46] The workshops followed-on from previous consultations held between 1987 and 1990 and were a response to indications from every province that public concerns raised in EIAs were increasingly related to health and the quality of life.

The workshops recommended that:

- health should be included in the scoping process although detailed health assessments may not be required for every project;
- the assessment should include socio-cultural effects on health and well-being as well as occupational health;
- health professionals had a vital role to play in EIA and were trusted by communities, but needed to collaborate more strongly with EIA professionals;
- health professionals should accept the constraints of the EIA process with regard to time, resources and scope and should provide clear and consistent advice;
- improved baseline data on community health, socio-cultural health and well-being were required and these, in turn, would require scientific strengthening of indicators;
- public participation was vital and better risk communication strategies were needed;
- policies, programmes and plans should be included as well as projects;
- health should be included by up-grading skills of existing professionals rather than by seeking additional resources;

- national guidance materials should be produced;
- incorporating health in EIA was a preventive health measure that would be cost-effective in the long-term.

The workshops also emphasised that the determinants of health included:
- income and social status;
- social support networks;
- education;
- employment and working conditions;
- physical environments;
- biology and genetic endowment;
- personal health practices and coping skills;
- healthy child development; and health services.

These determinants formed the basis for a proposed National Accord on Health and Environment that was consistent with health impact assessment. A questionnaire was circulated to several hundred professionals and there was strong agreement on many factors, including the need to incorporate occupational health and safety in health impact assessment.

A draft of a "National health guide for environmental assessment" was issued in 1995.[47] The guide aimed to assist health professionals to fulfill their growing obligations to participate in the EIA process: "health professionals unaware of the environmental assessment framework or processes, are being called upon to contribute their health expertise to the environmental assessment". It also aimed to contribute to the development of a scientific approach to HIA and to consider the data and information needs for scientific, political, public and legislative purposes. It set out a series of principles and provided checklists for including health in the screening and EIA stages. It included concerns for psycho-social well-being as well as physical health and emphasised public participation. It also referred to the need for the assessment of policies and programmes — "broad environmental and health issues that should have been addressed earlier when policies were developed surface during the assessment of a specific project, slowing down and complicating the assessment process".

The linkage between economic well-being and health was noted: "communities with adequate incomes can afford to eat more balanced diets and to live more healthy lifestyles".

The Canadian Guide identifies the same components of community vulnerability, environment and capability of health protection agencies. It tends to focus on pollution and chemical hazards. There are repeated references to psycho-social well-being but without specific examples of how this could be determined or safeguarded.

The European Union: recent developments

EC legislation relating to environmental impact assessment is discussed in Chapter 3. The information in this section derives from the University of Manchester, EIA Centre Newsletter.[48] The EIA Centre was established in January 1988 to organise and develop future EIA activities. The newsletter is prepared with financial support from the European Commission, Directorate-General XI - Environment, Nuclear Safety and Civil Protection, Nature Protection and Soil Conservation (XI.B.2).

Austria

The Federal Ministry of the Environment, Youth and Family Affairs and the competent authorities have established a working group to discuss recent developments and problems in the field of EIA. This group is an important forum for the ongoing exchange of information and has also been used for teaching and training purposes. As Austrian EIA legislation is currently being reviewed to take account of the new EIA Directive, the working group has divided into technical and legal sub-groups which aim to discuss and develop a draft revision of the Austrian EIA law. The Federal Ministry of the Environment, Youth and Family Affairs commissioned a study on strategic environmental assessment (SEA) which has been published (in German).[49] The Ministry is also taking part in a pilot project on strategic environmental assessment.

Belgium

Amendments have recently been made to the way in which EIA initiatives are supervised in the Brussels Capital Region.[50,51] EIA initiatives were previously supervised by the Brussels Institute for Environmental Management; under the new laws, major infrastructure projects, buildings and certain land use plans will be subject to an EIA under the supervision of the Brussels Regional Administration for Urban Development.

The first EIA guideline books for Flanders have been prepared with the assistance of the University of Antwerp. The guidelines set standards for good practice and, in addition to dealing with procedural and methodological aspects, they provide recommendations on how to conduct EIA for various disciplines. A study on the development of a user-friendly methodology for EIA for policies, plans and programmes for Flanders, conducted by the Vrije Universiteit Brussels, is expected to be concluded by the end of 1997.

Denmark

Although some improvements have been made to the project-level EIA process in Denmark (such as the requirement for public participation during the scoping phase), a pilot study on EIA quality undertaken by the EIA Centre at Roskilde University has found that EIS quality is generally far from satisfactory and that the EIA process as a whole should be subject to quality reviews.

A new provision for EIA of budgets was issued during 1997 and the environmental impact statement for the 1998 budget was presented in the Autumn. This approach is currently experimental and some difficulties, due to the focus being on separate activities, rather than the budget as a whole, have been identified. A study of EIA of a number of Danish policies has confirmed that assessment is integrated within the normal process of bill preparation within the ministries. However, the study showed that ministries tended to focus on positive rather than negative environmental effects and that systematic scoping techniques were not employed. The Ministry of Environment is currently reviewing the available guidance and methodological development activities.

Finland

So far, 90 projects have been subject to the Finnish EIA Act of 1994; these have included road projects, waste treatment facilities, power lines, power plants and peat production areas. Transboundary EIA is receiving attention and case study experience from Sweden and Russia has shown that the process of handling transboundary issues requires further development. The EIA guide for the Arctic was developed under the auspices of the Arctic Environmental Protection Strategy and approved by Arctic Ministers in 1997. Guidelines for the strategic assessment of plans, policies and programmes are due to be published by the Ministry of the Environment at the end of 1997. Further work is being undertaken into the environmental assessment of government bills.

France

The Ministry for Public Planning and the Environment (Amenagément du Territoire et Environnement) launched three working parties in 1997 which focused on the following areas: reinforcing the effectiveness and efficiency of EIA; reinforcing public participation during the EIA process; introducing the environmental assessment of policies, plans and programmes.

The working parties presented their conclusions at a one-day conference in Paris in September and a final report will be published. As a result of these activities, numerous proposals have been made to improve the EIA process in France, including:

- introducing scoping into the EIA process; creating more specific procedures;
- introducing a screening procedure to reduce the number of EIAs undertaken in France each year (presently between 5,000 and 6,000);
- organising public consultation prior to the public enquiry process;
- facilitating public participation during the public enquiry by improving the exchange of information;
- improving the competence of decision-makers, developers and consultants in charge of EIA;

- organising training for the public and non-governmental organisations
  (NGOs) so as to improve their knowledge of environmental protection and
  EIA procedures;
- improving the competence of the "commissaire enquêteur" (enquiry
  inspector) in charge of the public enquiry.

A number of members of the working parties believed that the proposals for an EU
Directive on strategic environmental assessment (SEA) should include policies as well as
plans and programmes.

A new commission, Commission Nationale du Débat Public (CNDP) was officially
launched in September 1997 by the Minister for Public Planning and the Environment. The
commission aims to encourage consultation relating to some projects and develop a
framework for effective consultation. The CNDP could ultimately become a means of
introducing public consultation within the strategic environmental assessment of national
transport schemes.

Germany

An official inquiry initiated by the opposition party has provided some data relating to the
state of EIA in Germany and the Federal States. As the Federal Government is responsible
for only a few EIAs, the Federal States were involved in the inquiry, although only a few
states were able to provide exact numbers of EIAs undertaken. Overall, the Federal
Government is satisfied with the current state of EIA practice.

A new planning act due to enter into force at the beginning of 1998 (Bau- und
Raumordnungsgesetz) includes changes to EIA as it applies to land use planning at the
municipal level and takes into account the amendments to the EIA Directive (97/11/EC).

The German government considered the proposal for a Council Directive on
strategic impact assessment[52] but expressed doubt as to whether new or additional
procedures were needed. The Bundesrat (representing the federal states) also voted
against the proposed directive on the grounds that:

- Experience should first be gained with the implementation of Directive
  97/11/EC.

- The Commission should apply SEA to its own programmes before introducing new requirements for the member states.
- Land use planning procedures would be burdened with additional requirements.
- As there is a delay between the development and implementation of plans and programmes, it is debatable whether project EIA would be made easier by SEA.
- The SEA proposal does not fit easily within the German planning system.
- The proposed procedures for public participation and transboundary consultation would lead to inefficiency and cost without environmental gain.

Further discussion among the various committees of the German parliament is planned.

Greece

A study is currently being undertaken by the Greek Ministry of Environmental and Public Works in association with the University of Thessalonika, the Technical Chamber of Greece and the private sector into the development of detailed specifications for undertaking impact assessments in accordance with the requirements of Directives 85/337/EEC and 97/11/EC. As a result of the study, a framework will be established to facilitate improvements in EIA practice such as: the development of detailed EIA requirements; the presentation of critical issues, and the exploration of mitigation measures.

Ireland

In Ireland, SEA is becoming a recognised means of advancing the integration of environmental considerations into key policy areas which provides a preventative rather than a remedial approach. The *Sustainable Development Strategy for Ireland*[53] sets out specific initiatives to bring forward proposals to develop an SEA system for major plans and programmes. This is in addition to supporting the EU proposals for the SEA of land use plans and programmes.

Italy

Several regions are undertaking legislative changes or developments to take account of the requirements of the Directive 97/11/EC and those of the proposed SEA Directive. These developments have sparked a renewed interested in EIA and a demand for EIA training with a strong practical orientation based on case study material.

The Netherlands

The second evaluation of the EIA process to have been undertaken since 1987 (when the system was introduced) will be concluded towards the end of 1997 and will be coupled with a response from the Government regarding the legislative aspects. Changes are expected to take place to accommodate the requirements of amendments to the EC Directive, relating primarily to the following areas:

- Strengthening the role of local government as a competent authority. Decision making will be transferred from the Ministry of the Environment in the majority of cases involving a request for exemption from EIA. The EIA Commission will, however, retain its advisory role.
- Applying EIA on a more selective basis by transferring certain activities from Annex I to Annex II.
- The selective application of post-decision follow-up. This represents a departure from the current requirement to undertake follow-up in all cases. The competent authority must determine, as part of the decision, whether an evaluation is required, and if so, for which aspects it should be performed and at what time. Enforcement measures will be implemented to promote compliance.
- Increased emphasis on the practical use of SEA as a tool for strategic decision-making within the current legal framework.

A further development is that several EIAs have led to increased pressure for changes in the methodology of impact prediction. This has become most apparent in relation to aircraft noise, airport safety, perception of noise, risks and air pollution from various activities. In the long term, improved EIA methodologies should lead to better standards for judging the environmental acceptability of a proposed activity.

Spain

Council Directive 85/337/EEC has been implemented in Spain through two national regulations and by subsequent legal provisions established by the Autonomous Communities. In order to overcome practice based deficiencies and to take into account the requirements of Directive 97/11/EC, Spanish EIA legislation is currently being reviewed. Some of the main features of the draft amendments are as follows:

- expanding the number of project types for which EIA is mandatory;
- establishing clear screening criteria, based on thresholds for noise, water and air quality;
- improving the scoping process;
- establishing a well-defined strategic environmental assessment procedure for plans and programmes;
- preliminary analysis of large scale alternatives in order to achieve more realistic project solutions during the early stages of the EIA process;
- developing transboundary EIA.

A number of SEAs have been undertaken in the communities. These mainly relate to land management issues. It is interesting to note that in contrast to many other EU members, the communities often make no overt recognition of the differences between plan, programme and project EIA procedures. Only the community of Castilla y Leon makes a clear distinction between EIA and SEA procedures.

USA

A review of the US experience concluded that health had been given minimal attention in most environmental impact assessments.[54] Considerable attention has been paid to assessing existing health risks in American cities using a procedure referred to as comparative risk assessment. This focuses primarily on chemical hazards and is concerned with frequency and severity of exposure. It has been extended by the United States Agency for International Development (USAID) to environmental health assessment in developing country cities.[55] Environmental health assessment is described as a combination of health risk assessment, health effects assessment and ethnographic investigation of health-related behaviour. It combines secondary data on environmental quality and the occurrence of environmentally related disease with primary ethnographic data collected by a field study team. The outputs of such studies could be relevant to the prospective assessment of new projects. The conclusions reached in one such study are illustrated in Table 11.

Risk score	Determinants of risk
High	Food contamination, outdoor air pollution
Medium	Traffic hazards, occupational hazards, drinking water, wastewater, indoor air pollution
Low	Solid waste, pesticide contamination of food
Not estimated	Lead in air, pesticides in non-food sources

Table 11: Assessment of environmental health risks in the city of Quito, Ecuador, (1993)[56]

Appendix 6

Coverage of impacts on human health in UK environmental impact statements: a review

Methodology

Thirty-nine environmental impact statements (EISs) for proposed developments in the UK were selected at random from a collection held by Oxford Brookes University, and they were reviewed to establish the extent and depth of their discussion of impacts on human health. The 39 EISs were all produced between 1988 and 1994 (inclusive) for a range of types of proposed developments; the 39 EISs are all listed at the end of this appendix. They included proposals for clinical waste incinerators, landfill sites, opencast coal mines, road improvements and bypasses, sewage treatment works, power stations and agricultural units. The magnitude and severity of the potential impacts on human beings and their health in those proposals varies between the different types of developments and between individual projects of the same broad type. It would have been unrealistic to have expected uniform coverage of health issues in the EISs, and therefore it is inevitably difficult to make direct comparisons. An attempt has been made, however, to summarise the coverage of health issues according to a set of common criteria, such as whether or not they:

- contained specific sections on issues of human health;
- referred to impacts on human health in non-technical summaries;
- assessed impacts on human health;
- included a characterisation of the 'receiving population';
- referred to the relevance of health considerations in site selection and project design;
- referred to consultation on health issues, particularly with health professionals; and
- adequately covered relevant issues of human health.

Results

Inclusion of specific sections on human health issues

The majority of the 39 EISs (72%) did not list in their tables of contents sections or chapters which explicitly discussed human health or related issues. Only 28% of the EISs, therefore, listed sections directly relevant to the assessment of impacts on human health. 13% of the EISs listed sections concerned with 'impacts on human beings and/or local communities', but they were not specifically related to health, and sections on 'safety' and/or 'hazards' were included in 15% of the EISs. Only one EIS included a section which made direct reference to human health in a chapter on 'exposure assessment — health effects'. 15% of the EISs contained appendices which related to human health issues. For example, one included a copy of the company's health and safety and environmental policies. A second example included appendices summarising the findings of toxicity and hazard operability studies. Other EISs included, as appendices, studies of noise disturbance and copies of the EC and WHO Air Quality Standards and Guidelines.

Reference to impacts on human health in non-technical summaries

The inclusion of a non-technical summary (NTS) in an EIS is a specific requirement of the Town and Country Planning (Assessment of Environmental Effects) Regulations 1988. This provision was intended to make the findings of an environmental impact statement (which are often complex, technical and bulky) accessible to non-specialist readers. Of the sample of 39 EISs, only 10 (26%) included a NTS, and of those, only 3 made direct reference to issues of human health or safety. This implies that not only do the majority of proponents fail to meet the specified regulatory requirements by failing to make EIS-findings accessible to the general public, but they place little emphasis on environmental health and safety as issues of public concern.

Assessment of impacts on human health

While few EISs devoted specific sections to issues of human health and/or safety, a number made reference to, or included some analysis of, impacts with potential health implications. 49% of the sample of EISs made no specific references whatever to human health. 28%

referred to public health and safety and to the health and safety of employees. With respect to occupational health and safety, 73% of the EISs which addressed this issue also included assessments of possible impacts and some indication of proposed mitigation measures. In relation to public health and safety, only 45% analysed potential impacts in any depth. Only 5% of these EISs included detailed assessments of potential impacts on public health, estimating likely uptakes of pollutants by people and some of their effects. One of these, for example, explored the possible links between dust and asthma. Another EIS discussed the results of toxicity tests intended to establish the safety or toxicity of the wastes expected to arise; the tests were conducted on rats, and estimated uptake figures for the public were not provided. Other possible indirect impacts were sometimes discussed. Table 12 lists the 13 types of impacts, and indicates the percentage of the EISs in which those impacts were discussed.

While all these factors can have implications for health, this was rarely made explicit in this sample of EISs. The potential impact on public health of the predicted levels of noise or air pollution were not discussed or analysed. In those cases in which levels of noise were assessed, the discussion was in terms of volume in particular locations rather than in terms of the likely effects on people, such as their preferences or tolerances of such disturbance, or the likely disruption of patterns of sleep. As a general rule, the information provided in the EISs was insufficient to predict actual health impacts, because the affected population was rarely characterised.

Only one of the EISs that predicted emissions of dust discussed possible links between that dust and an aspect of human health, namely asthma. Similarly, in relation to air pollution, only one EIS attempted to model patterns of the deposition of those pollutants and estimated the possible implications for the release of carcinogenic materials to the local inhabitants. In other cases, the tendency was for the EIS merely to focus on the issue of compliance with environmental quality standards or emission limits. The problem with that approach is that cumulative effects may be neglected, because compliance with standards or limits does not take account of longterm exposure to the pollutant.

Characterisation of receiving population

Sixty-seven percent of the sample of EISs included no information which would have made it possible to estimate the size of population likely to be affected, while 21% provided some

Types of impact	% of EISs including the impact
Noise	62
Air pollution	59
Traffic	44
Water pollution	38
Dust	31
Odour	18
Loss of amenity	13
Vermin	10
Negative social impacts (eg severance of communities)	10
Vibration	8
Positive social impacts (eg reduced unemployment)	8
Disruption of contaminated ground (eg release of toxic dust)	8
Animal diseases (eg of farm livestock)	5

limited information, typically estimates of the size of the local population. Only 13% gave any estimates of the population likely to be affected by the potential impacts of the proposed projects. The majority of those 13% (60% of them) did this only with respect to the effects of noise. None of the 39 EISs categorised affected populations according to their likely vulnerability to potential adverse impacts on health. This highlights the absence of any systematic or detailed assessments of health impacts, because without characterising the 'receiving population', it is impossible to predict the health impacts of any proposal.

Role of health considerations in site selection and project design

Only 18% of the 39 EISs mentioned health or public safety as having influenced site selection or project design. In most of those cases, such references were brief; one for example said that: "proximity of occupied properties was a factor in determining the sensitivity of the proposed location". In two cases (5% of the EISs), enhanced safety was cited as one objective of the proposals. For example, improved road safety as grounds for widening a road.

Consultation

The majority of the 39 EISs indicated that the developers had consulted with statutory consultees concerning their proposals, and with others, but a substantial majority (62%) provided no evidence of any consultation in relation to human health. 18% of the EISs indicated that consultation had taken place with local environmental health departments and 8% reported consulting with public health departments (in Scotland). 23% recorded consultation with (what then was) Her Majesty's Inspectorate of Pollution (now part of the Environment Agency) and 18% with the Health and Safety Executive. There was one report of consultation with a Public Health and Safety Inspector. The evidence clearly shows that consultation with health professionals, environmental health departments and the Health and Safety Executive was not a routine event for new proposed developments.

Adequacy of coverage of health issues

There was little consistency in the reported coverage of health-related issues in the 39 cases examined. The information in the sample of EISs suggests that the potential adverse health effects of proposed developments were adequately covered in approximately 28% of cases. The evidence suggested that public health issues were generally addressed more comprehensively in relation to 5 of the 39 developments which fell under Schedule 1 of the UK Town and Planning Regulations. Even in those cases, however, the extent to which considerations of public health were addressed was not necessarily as substantial as might have been hoped for, given the scale and severity of potential problems.

Conclusions

While the legislation which refers to Environmental Assessments has created an opportunity for the public health consequences of environmental changes to be addressed, most participants, ie developers and their environmental consultants, clearly have not regarded those aspects as important or even worthy of consideration. Some of the 39 EISs which were reviewed indicated that they could pose potentially significant hazards for human health, but in the majority of cases the EISs failed to provide due consideration of those matters. There was, in general, a failure to provide the information which would be required by anyone wanting to assess the likely implications of the proposed development for human health. The populations and the types of individuals likely to be affected by proposed developments were rarely identified. Their likely exposure and probable impacts were rarely estimated and their relative vulnerabilities were not discussed. Social impacts were largely neglected and there was little effort to gauge or evaluate the opinions and wishes of the local people.

There is no clear procedure which developers, their consultants and public officials can follow when assessing the implications for public health of developmental proposals. There is, therefore, an evident risk that developments, as currently assessed, might exert adverse effects on public health, either individually or cumulatively.

There are a number of possible explanations for the lack of emphasis given to issues of environmental health and safety in the sample of 39 environmental impact statements these include:

- the EISs reviewed were for developments unlikely to have significant impacts on health;
- the proponents wished to downplay and understate potential impacts on health;
- assessing human health impacts is complex and would require incurring currently avoidable costs;
- the legislation fails explicitly to require an assessment of the implications for public and occupational health;
- there are no clear procedures or methodologies for assessing the health implications of new developments.

The evidence provided by this study is not sufficient to establish the extent to which those various considerations contribute to providing an explanation of the shortcomings which have been uncovered and outlined. Further studies of larger samples in greater detail will help to clarify these important issues.

Environmental impact statements (1988-94) reviewed •

1988	Landfill site, Seghill.
1988	Wallingford Bypass.
1989	Construction and operation of a clinical waste disposal unit at a sewage treatment works, Tyne and Wear.
1989	Grass landing strip and associated maintenance facility, Wilts.
1989	Neutralised digester residues: filtration and disposal, Grimsby.
1989	North West ethylene pipeline.
1990	Birmingham airport link pipeline.
1990	Crude oil export facilities, Dalmeny and Hound.
1990	Regional Sewage Disposal Scheme, Teign Estuary.
1990	Sheffield and Rotherham City Airport.
1991	Clinical waste Incinerator Installations, Shotts.
1991	Clinical waste incinerator, Dundee.
1991	Clinical waste incinerator, Knostrop.
1991	Intermediate level nuclear waste store, Sellafield.
1991	Veterinary waste incinerator, Devon.
1992	A53 Hodnet Bypass.
1992	Disposal of controlled wastes by landfill, Watnall.
1992	Quarry-infill, Ugley.
1992	Replacement incinerator plant, Portsmouth.
1993	Disposal of special waste by landfilling, Grimsby.
1993	Forge and Monument Restoration Scheme.
1993	Manchester Airport Second Runway.
1993	Redhill Aerodrome.
1993	Sewage treatment, Taw Torridge, N. Area.
1993	Terminal 5, Heathrow Airport.

1993	Turkey farm, Freiston.
1994	B4031 road improvements.
1994	M5 widening, junctions 18 to 19.
1994	Residential and marina development.
1994	Waste disposal site, Hants.
Date not specified	Clinical waste incinerator, Redditch.
Date not specified	Opencast coal site, Airdsgreen.
Date not specified	Poultry unit.
Date not specified	Power Station, Peterborough.
Date not specified	Proposed development for scrap tyre burning, Grantham.
Date not specified	Railway vehicle operation (asbestos development), Desford.
Date not specified	Selar Opencast Project.
Date not specified	Sizewell 'C', nuclear electric power station.
Date not specified	Worcester Western Bypass.

References

Chapter 1

1 British Medical Association. *Pesticides, chemicals and health*. London: Edward Arnold, 1992

2 British Medical Association. *Road transport and health*. London: BMA, 1997

3 British Medical Association. *Complementary medicine: new approaches to good practice*. Oxford: Oxford University Press, 1993

4 British Medical Association. *Code of practice for the safe use and disposal of sharps*. London: BMA, 1995

5 British Medical Association. *Environmental and occupational risks of health care*. London: BMA, 1994

6 British Medical Association. *The BMA guide to living with risk*. London: Penguin Books, 1990

7 See reference 1

8 British Medical Association. *Hazardous waste and human health*. Oxford: Oxford University Press, 1991

9 British Medical Association. *Cycling: towards health and safety*. Oxford: Oxford University Press, 1992

10 See reference 2

11 British Medical Association. *Water: a vital resource*. London: BMA, 1994

12 See reference 5

13 See reference 4

14 British Medical Association. *A Code of practice for sterilisation of instruments and control of cross infection*. London: BMA, 1995

15 See reference 8

16 British Medical Association. *Inequalities in health*. London: BMA, 1995

17 Environmental Health Commission. *Agendas for change*. London: Chartered Institute for Environmental Health, 1997

18 Proposal for a Council Directive on the assessment of the effects of certain plans and programmes on the environment. COM/96/0511 Final - Syn 96/0304. *Official Journal of the European Communities*. No C129,25/4/97

19 Commission of the European Communities. *Report from the Commission to the Council, the European Parliament and the Economic and Social Committee on the integration of health protection in community policies*. COM/95/196 Final 29 May 1995. Brussels: CEC, 1995

Chapter 2

1 Royal Commission on Environmental Pollution. *10th Report*. London: HMSO, 1984

2 British Medical Association. *The medical effects of nuclear war. The report of the British Medical Association's Board of Science and Education*. London: BMA, 1983

3 Gilpin A. *Environmental impact assessment: cutting edge for the twenty first century*. Cambridge: Cambridge University Press, 1995

4 Department of the Environment. *Sustainable development: The UK strategy*. London: HMSO, 1994

5 See reference 3

6 World Commission on Environment and Development. *Our common future*. Oxford: Oxford University Press, 1988

7 United Nations. *The global partnership for environment and development, a guide to Agenda 21 post Rio edition*. New York: United Nations, 1993

8 Birley MH and Peralta GL. Health impact assessment of development projects. In: Vanclay F and Bronstein DA, eds. *Social and environmental impact assessment*. New York: Wiley and Sons, 1996

9 British Medical Association. *Environmental and occupational risks of health care*. London: BMA, 1994

10 Chartered Institute of Environmental Health. *Environmental health for sustainable development*. London: CIEH, 1995

11 Department of the Environment. *The British Government Panel on sustainable development. Third report*. London: HMSO, 1997

12 See reference 4

13 See reference 9

14 McMichael AJ. *Planetary overload. Global environmental change and the health of the human species*. Cambridge: Cambridge University Press, 1993

15 World Health Organisation Office of Global and Integrated Environmental Health (programme editor McMichael, AJ). *Climate change and human health: An assessment prepared by a task group on behalf of the WHO, WMO and UNEP*. Geneva: WHO, 1996

16 Department of the Environment and the Department of Health. *The United Kingdom National Environmental Health Action Plan*. Cm 3323. London: HMSO, 1996

17 See reference 15

18 World Health Organisation. *European Charter on environment and health*. Copenhagen: WHO Regional Office for Europe, 1989

19 See reference 16

20 Department of the Environment, Transport and the Regions. *Green Ministers get down to business*. 312/ENV. 30 Jul 1997

21 Department of the Environment, Transport and the Regions. *Green Ministers set out Whitehall agenda for action*. 315/ENV. 31 Jul 1997

22   Department of Health. *The Health of the Nation. A strategy for health in England*. London: HMSO, 1992

23   Department of Health. *Our Healthier Nation*: Green Paper. London: HMSO, 1998

24   Department of Health and Department of the Environment. *Consultative Document - The environment and health*. 96DPL 0022. London: HMSO, 1996

25   Department of Health. *Health of the Nation: fit for the future*. London: HMSO, 1995a

26   Department of Health. *Health of the Nation: variations in health*. London: HMSO, 1995b

27   See reference 23

28   See reference 23

29   Department of Health. *Ministerial appointments for health announced and responsibilities allocated*. Press release 97/090, 1997

30   Olsen N. At last, a public health minister. *BMJ* 1997;314:1498-99

31   See reference 16

32   Environment Agency. *An environmental strategy for the millennium and beyond*. Bristol: EA, 1997

33   See reference 16

34   Department of Health. *On the state of the public health: The Annual Report of the Chief Medical Officer of The Department of Health for the Year 1996*. London: HMSO, 1997

35   NHS Management Executive. *Public health: responsibilities of the NHS and the roles of others. Advice of the Committee set up to review of HC(88)64. Issued with Health Service Guidelines HSG(93)56*. Leeds: NHS Management Executive, 1993

36   Buckinghamshire Health Authority. *Annual Report from the Director of Public Health*. Aylesbury. Buckinghamshire Health Authority, 1996

37   See reference 9

38   See reference 34

39   Department of Health. *The New NHS*: White Paper. Cm 3807. London: HMSO, 1997

40   See reference 16

41   Environmental Health Commission. *Agendas for change*. London: Chartered Institute of Environmental Health, 1997

42   Stein A. Government and legislative control of environmental hazards - private sector. In *Oxford Textbook of Public Health (1st Edn) Volume 1*. Oxford: Oxford University Press, 1984:154-160.

43   See reference 42

44   O'Riordan T, Cameron J, eds. *Interpreting the precautionary principle*. London: Earthscan, 1994

45   Department of the Environment. *This common inheritance. Britain's environmental strategy*. Cm 1200. London: HMSO, 1990

46   See reference 16

47   See reference 42

48   See reference 42

49   Adapted from White PR, De Smet B, Owens JW, Hindel P. Environmental management in an international consumer goods company. *Resources, Conservation and Recycling* 1995;14:171-184

50   See reference 49

51   Von Zharen WM. *ISO 14000: Understanding the environmental standards*. Maryland, USA: Government Institutes Inc., 1996

52   European Public Health Alliance. *Public health and the EU - an overview*. Brussels: EPHA, 1995

53   Commission of the European Communities. *Report from the Commission to the Council, the European Parliament and the Economic and Social Committee on the integration of health protection in community policies*. COM/95/196 Final 29 May 1995. Brussels: CEC, 1995

54   Rayner M. European Union policy and health. *BMJ* 1995;311:1180-1181

55   See reference 16

56   See reference 16

57   Department of Health. *Policy appraisal and health, a guide for policy makers*. London: HMSO, 1995

58   See reference 41

59   Wood C. *Environmental impact assessment: A comparative review*. Harlow, Essex: Longman, 1995

60   Adetona OO. *The treatment of human health impacts within environmental impact assessment*. MSc Thesis, University of Manchester, Department of Environmental Biology, 1995

Chapter 3

1   Department of the Environment. *Environmental assessment: A guide to the procedures*. London: HMSO, 1989

2   Council Directive 97/11/EC of 3 March 1997 amending Directive 85/337/EEC on the assessment of the effects of certain public and private projects on the environment. *Official Journal of the European Communities*. No L073,14/3/97

3   See reference 1

4   Council Directive 85/337/EEC of 27 June 1985 on the assessment of the effects of certain public and private projects on the environment. *Official Journal of the European Communities*. No L176,5/7/85

5   See reference 2

6   Vanclay F, Bronstein D, eds. *Environmental and social impact assessment*. Chichester: Wiley, 1995

7   Glasson J, Therivel R, Chadwick A. *Introduction to environmental impact assessment: Principles and procedures, process, practice and prospects. The natural and built environment: Series 1*. London: University College London Press, 1994

8   Therivel R, Wilson E, Thompson S, Heaney D, Pritchard D. *Strategic environmental assessment*. London: Earthscan Publications Ltd, 1992

9   Proposal for a Council Directive on the assessment of the effects of certain plans and programmes on the environment. COM/96/0511 Final - Syn 96/0304. *Official Journal of the European Communities*. No C129,25/4/97

10   Sadler B, Baxter M. Taking Stock of SEA. *Environmental Assessment* 1997;5:14-16

11   See reference 9

12   Tsoskounoglou E. Social Environmental Impact Assessment: A tool for community sensitive and sustainable development. *Environmental Assessment* 1997;5:20-22

13   Carley MJ and Bustelo ES. *Social impact assessment and monitoring: a guide to the literature*. Boulder, Colorado: Westview Press, 1984

14   Gilpin A. *Environmental Impact Assessment: Cutting edge for the twenty first century*. Cambridge: Cambridge University Press, 1995

15   See reference 14

16   See reference 12

17   Layfield, Frank, Sir. *Sizewell B public inquiry*. London: HMSO, 1987

18   See reference 7

19   British Medical Association. *Inequalities in health*. London: BMA, 1995

20   See reference 12

21   World Health Organisation. *Health and safety component of environmental impact assessment. Environmental Health Series No.15*. Copenhagen: WHO Regional Office for Europe, 1987

22   Birley MH, Peralta GL. Health impact assessment of development projects. In: Vanclay F, Bronstein DA, eds. *Social and environmental impact assessment*. New York: Wiley and Sons, 1996

23   Adetona OO. *The treatment of human health impacts within environmental impact assessment*. MSc Thesis, University of Manchester, Department of Environmental Biology, 1995

24   See reference 4

25   See reference 2

26   See reference 4

27   Department of the Environment Circular 15/88 (Welsh Office 23/88): *Environmental assessment* - 12 July 1988

28   Department of Transport, Scottish Office, Welsh Office, Department of Environment Northern Ireland. *Volume 11. Design manual for roads and bridges*. Second edition. London: HMSO, 1994

29   See reference 2

30   Department of the Environment, Transport and the Regions. *Environmental Assessment: Implementation of EC Directive (97/11/EC) on Environmental Assessment*. London: DETR, July 1997

31 Department of the Environment, Transport and the Regions. Implementation of EC Directive 97/11/EC: *Determining the need for environmental assessment*. London: DETR, December 1997

32 See reference 9

33 See reference 9

34 See reference 4

35 See reference 2

36 Department of the Environment. *DoE Circular 7/94 (Welsh Office 20/94): Environmental Assessment: Amendment of the Regulations*. London: HMSO, 1994

37 See reference 2

38 See reference 31

39 See reference 4

40 See reference 2

41 See reference 2

42 See reference 1

43 See reference 28

44 Department of the Environment. *The United Kingdom National Air Quality Strategy. Cm 3587*. London: HMSO, 1997

45 See reference 1

46 National Centre for Risk Analysis and Options Appraisal. *Road transport and the environment. Risk Profile No 1*. London: Environment Agency, 1997

Chapter 4

1 Sadler B. *International study of effectiveness of environmental assessment*. Canadian Environmental Assessment Agency and the International Association for Impact Assessment, 1996

2 Wjst M, Reitmeir P, Dold S, Wulff A, Nicolai T, von Loeffelholz-Xolberg E, von Matius E. Road traffic and adverse effects on respiratory health in children. *British Medical Journal* 1993;307:596-600

3 British Medical Association. *The BMA guide to living with risk*. London: Penguin Books, 1990

4 Department of Health. *On the state of the public health, the Annual Report of the Chief Medical Officer of the Department of Health for the year 1996*. London: HMSO, 1997

5 Brown V, Smith DI, Wiseman R, Handmer J. *Risks and opportunities: Managing environmental conflict and change*. London: Earthscan, 1995

6 Council Directive 85/337/EEC of 27 June 1985 on the assessment of the effects of certain public and private projects on the environment. *Official Journal of the European Communities*. No L176,5/7/85

7 Town and Country Planning (Assessment of Environmental Effects) Regulations 1988 (SI No. 1199)

8   Department of the Environment Circular 15/88 (Welsh Office 23/88): *Environmental assessment* - 12 July 1988

9   See reference 8

10   See reference 8

11   Scottish Development Department Circular 13/88: *Environmental assessment: Implementation of the EC Directive: The Environmental Assessment (Scotland) Regulations 1988* - 12 July 1988

12   Department of the Environment (Northern Ireland): *Development Control Advice Note 10*

13   Department of the Environment, Transport and the Regions. Implementation of EC Directive 97/11/EC: *Determining the need for environmental assessment.* London: DETR, December 1997

14   See reference 13

15   Morgan DR, ed. *Managing biological and chemical risks'.* London: Institute of Biology, 1997

16   Office of Population Census and Survey. Health Statistics Unit. *Unpublished data,* 1996

17   Council Directive 97/11/EC of 3 March 1997 amending Directive 85/337/EEC on the assessment of the effects of certain public and private projects on the environment. *Official Journal of the European Communities.* No L073,14/3/97

18   Department of the Environment, Transport and the Regions. *Environmental Assessment: Implementation of EC Directive (97/11/EC) on Environmental Assessment.* London: DETR, July 1997

19   Environment Agency. *Environmental assessment: Scoping handbook for projects.* London: HMSO 1996

20   British Medical Association. *Pesticides, chemicals and health.* London: Edward Arnold, 1992

21   Cooper Weil DEC, Alicbusan AP, Wilson JF, Reich MR and Bradley DJ. *The impact of development policies on health: A review of the literature.* Geneva: WHO, 1990

22   Bradley D, Stephens C, Harpham T, Cairncross S. *A review of environmental health impacts in developing country cities.* Urban Management Program Discussion Paper 6. Washington: The World Bank, 1992

23   Birley MH. *The health impact assessment of development projects.* London: HMSO, 1995

24   See reference 23

25   British Medical Association. *Environmental and occupational risks of health care.* London: BMA, 1994

26   Public Health Laboratory Service. Multiple Drug Resistant Staphylococcus aureus (MRSA). *Communicable Disease Report* May 1997;7:22

27   Anon. Revised guidelines for the control of epidemic methicillin-resistant Staphylococcus aureus. Report of a combined working party of the Hospital Infection Society and British Society for Antimicrobial Chemotherapy. *Journal of Hospital Infection* Nov 1990;16:351-77

28   Lessing, MPA. When should healthcare workers be screened for methicillin-resistant Staphylococcus aureus? *Journal of Hospital Infection* 1996;3:197-303

29   Cox RA, Conquest C. Strategies for the management of healthcare staff colonized with epidemic methicillin-resistant Staphylococcus aureus. *Journal of Hospital Infection* 1997;2:117-127

30   Letters to the editor. *Journal of Hospital Infection* 1997;4

31 Correspondence. *British Medical Journal* 1997;315:57-60

32 Public Health Laboratory Service. *Vero cytotoxin-producing Escherichia coli 0157*. Factsheet. London: PHLS, 15 Jan 1997

33 See reference 20

34 Ministry of Agriculture, Fisheries and Food. *The Food Standards Agency: A force for change*. Cm 3830. London: HMSO, 1998

35 Parliamentary Office of Science and Technology. *Breathing in our cities*. London: POST, 1994

36 Department of Health. *Asthma and outdoor air pollution*. London: HMSO, 1995

37 Lercher P, Schmitzberger R, Kofler W. Perceived traffic air pollution, associated behaviour and health in an alpine area. *Science of the Total Environment* 1995;169:71-74

38 Edward J, Walters S, Griffiths R. Hospital admissions for asthma in preschool children: relationship to major roads in Birmingham, United Kingdom. *Archives of Environmental Health* 1994;49:223-227

39 Weiland S, Mundt K, Ruckmann S, Keil U. Self-reported wheezing and allergic rhinitis in children and traffic density on street of residence. *Annals of Epidemiology* 1994;4:243-247

40 Department of Health. Committee on the Medical Effects of Air Pollutants. *Quantification of the effects of air pollution on health in the UK*. London: HMSO, 1998

41 Nutrition Task Force Low Income Project Team. *Low income, food, nutrition and health: strategies for improvement*. London: Department of Health, 1996

42 Department of Health. *Our Healthier Nation*: Green Paper. London: HMSO, 1998

43 See reference 34

44 Frankel S, Gunnell D, Peters J, Maynard M, Davey-Smith G. Childhood energy intake and adult mortality from cancer: the Boyd Orr cohort study. *BMJ* 1998;316:499- 504

45 Department of Transport. *Road casualties Great Britain: Final figures 1996*. London: HMSO, 1997

46 Sabey B. *Road safety into the 80s, symposium: recent developments and research in road safety remedial measures*. Manchester: University of Salford, 1983

47 Carson O, Tight M, Southwell M, Plows B. *Urban accidents: why do they happen?* Basingstoke: Automobile Association Foundation for Road Safety Research, 1990

48 Ohrstrom E. Psycho-social effects of traffic noise exposure. *Journal of Sound and Vibration* 1991;151:513-517

49 Institute of Environmental Health Officers. *Transportation: The route to health report*. London: IEHO, 1993

50 Kobayashi F, Furui H, Akamatsu Y, Natanabe T, Horibe H. Changes in psychophysiological functions during night shift in nurses. Influence of changing from a full day to a half day work-shift before night duty. *International Archives of Occupational and Environmental Health*. 1997;69:83-90

51 Rosen JC, Compass BE, Tacy B. The relation among stress, psychological symptoms and eating disorder symptoms: a prospective analysis. *International Journal of Eating Disorders* 1993;14:153-62

52 See reference 42

53   Prescott-Clarke P, Primatesta P, eds. *Health survey for England 1995: findings: a survey carried out on behalf of the Department of Health*. Series HS; No 5; vol 1. London: HMSO, 1997

54   Lowry S. *Housing and health*. London: British Medical Journal, 1991

55   See reference 42

56   Shuval HI. *Wastewater irrigation in developing countries: Health effects and technical solutions*. Water and Sanitation Discussion Paper Series, No 2. Washington: The International Bank for Reconstruction and Development, 1990

57   Shuval HI, et al. *Wastewater irrigation in developing countries: Health effects and technical solutions*. Washington: World Bank, 1986

58   See reference 6

59   See reference 17

60   Smith A. Scoping, public participation and the consultation process. *Environmental Assessment* 1997;5:36-38

61   Health and Safety (Emissions to the Atmosphere) Regulations 1983 (SI No.943)

62   Department of the Environment. *Environmental assessment. A guide to the procedures*. London: HMSO, 1989

63   See reference 17

64   See reference 13

65   See reference 20

66   British Medical Association. *Hazardous waste and human health*. Oxford: Oxford University Press, 1991

67   British Medical Association. *Inequalities in health*. London: BMA, 1995

68   See reference 66

69   See reference 20

70   See reference 3

71   See reference 25

72   See reference 66

73   See reference 25

74   See reference 4

75   Anon. *National health guide for environmental assessment: a discussion paper*. Prepared for the Federal-Provincial-Territorial Committee on Environmental and Occupational Health. The Environmental Health Centre. Ottawa: Health Canada, 1995

76   See reference 3

77   Critchley M, MacNalty A. *Butterworths Medical Dictionary Second Edition*. London: Butterworths, 1984

78   *Concise Encylopedia of Science and Technology*. Ed: S.P. Pancer, 2nd Edition. New York: McGraw-Hill
      Publishing, 1989

79   World Health Organisation. *Concern for Europe's tomorrow: Health and the environment in the WHO
      European region*. WHO European Centre for Environment and Health. Stuttgart: Wissenschaftliche
      Verlagsgesellschaft, 1995

80   See reference 25

81   See reference 79

82   Royal Commission on Environmental Pollution. *12th Report*. London: HMSO, 1988

83   McMurray J. *Organic chemistry 4th edition*. USA: Brooks H. Cole Publishing Company, 1996

84   Department of the Environment. *The United Kingdom national air quality strategy*. Cm 3587. London:
      HMSO, 1997

85   Air Quality Regulations 1997 (SI No. 3043)

86   See reference 40

87   Dockery DW, Pope CA 3rd. Environmental epidemiology program, Harvard School of Public Health, Boston,
      MA acute respiratory effects of particulate air pollution. *Annual Review of Public Health* 1994;15:107-32

88   See reference 40

89   Hansard. *Written answers*. 10 February 1998. WA166. London: HMSO, 1998

90   See reference 40

91   Wood C. *Environmental impact assessment: A comparative review*. Harlow, Essex: Longman, 1995

92   See reference 20

93   See reference 66

94   O'Riordan T, Cameron J, eds. *Interpreting the precautionary principle*. London: Earthscan, 1994

95   Department of the Environment. *This common inheritance. Britain's environmental strategy*. Cm 1200.
      London: HMSO, 1990

96   See reference 3

97   See reference 75

98   Covello VT, McCallum DB, Pavlova M. *Effective risk communication*. New York: Blenheim Press, 1989

99   See reference 3

100   See reference 4

101   See reference 7

102   Lee N, Colley R. *Reviewing environmental statements. Occasional paper No. 24*. EIA Centre, University of
      Manchester, 1990

103   See reference 25

104 Department of Health and Department of the Environment. *Public Health: responsibilities of the NHS and the roles of others. Advice of the committee set up to undertake a review of HC (88)64.* London: DH/DoE, 1993

105 Haddon W. Advances in the epidemiology of injuries as a basis for public policy. *Landmarks in American Epidemiology* 1980;95:411-421

106 See reference 75

107 Department of the Environment, Transport and the Regions. *Mitigation measures in environmental statements.* London: DETR, 1997

108 Mitchell J. Mitigation in environmental assessment: furthering best practice. *Environmental Assessment* 1997;5:28-29

109 See reference 75

110 See reference 75

111 Carley M. *Social measurements and social indicators: issues of policy and theory.* London: Allen and Unwin, 1981

112 Department of Health and Department of the Environment. *Consultative Document - The environment and health 96DPL 0022.* London: HMSO, 1996

113 See reference 42

114 British Medical Association. *Road transport and health.* London: BMA, 1997

115 Will S, Ardern K, Spencely M, Watkins S. *A prospective health impact assessment of the proposed development of a second runway at Manchester International Airport.* Written submission to the Public Inquiry. Manchester and Stockport Health Commissions, 1994

116 Teesside Environmental Epidemiology Study Group. *Health, illness and the environment in Teesside and Sunderland.* University of Newcastle: Departments of Epidemiology and Public Health and Social Policy, 1995

117 Moffatt S, Phillimore P, Bhopal R, Foy C. If this is what it's doing to our washing what is it doing to our lungs? Industrial pollution and public understanding in North-West England. *Social Science and Medicine* 1995;41:883-91

118 Department of the Environment and the Department of Health. *The United Kingdom National Environmental Health Action Plan.* Cm 3323. London: HMSO, 1996

119 Aberg N, Sundell J, Eriksson B, Hesselmar B, Aberg B. Prevalence of allergic disease in school children in relation to family history, upper respiratory infections, and residential characteristics. *Allergy* 1996;51:232-7

120 Tumwesigire SG, Barton T. Environmental risk factors of acute respiratory infections among children of military personnel in Uganda. *East Africa Medical Journal* 1995;72:290-4

121 Building Research Establishment. *Indoor air quality in homes. The Building Research Establishment Indoor Environment Study Parts 1 and 2 (Ref BR 299 and BR 300).* London: BRE, 1996

122 See reference 3

123 Hughes JS, O'Riordan MC. *Radiation exposure of the UK population - 1993 review.* R263. Oxford: National Radiological Protection Board, 1993

124   See reference 112

125   See reference 42

126   See reference 25

127   See reference 67

128   British Medical Association. *Strategies for national renewal: A British Medical Association commentary on the report of the commission on social justice*. London: BMA, 1996

129   Health and Safety Executive. *The costs to the British economy of work accidents and work-related ill health*. London: Health and Safety Executive, 1994

130   deCarteret J C. Occupational stress claims: effects on workers' compensation. *American Association of Occupational Health Nurses Journal* 1994;42:494-8

131   Hurrell JJ Jr, Murphy LR. Occupational stress intervention. *American Journal of Industrial Medicine* 1996;29:338-41

132   British Medical Association. *Stress and the medical profession*. London: BMA, 1992

133   British Medical Association. *The misuse of alcohol and other drugs by doctors*. London: BMA, 1998

134   Department of Health. *On the state of the public health, the Annual Report of the Chief Medical Officer of the Department of Health for the year 1994*. London: HMSO, 1995

135   Friends of the Earth. *Prescription for change: Health and the environment. Discussion paper 2*. London: FOE, 1995

136   See reference 75

137   Watt GCM. Health implications of putting value added tax on fuel. *BMJ* 1994;309:1030-31

138   Department of Transport. *Transport statistics Great Britain*. London: HMSO, 1995

139   See reference 45

140   Edwards J, Walters S, Griffiths R. Hospital admissions for asthma in preschool children: Relationship to major roads in Birmingham, United Kingdom. *Archives of Environmental Health* 1994;49:223-227

141   See reference 39

142   See reference 48

143   See reference 49

144   Lercher P, Kofler W. Behavioural and health responses associated with road traffic noise exposure along alpine through traffic routes. *Science of the Total Environment* 1996;89/190:85-89

145   Berkman L, Syme L. Social networks, host resistance and mortality: A nine year follow up study of Alameda County residents. *American Journal of Epidemiology* 1979;109:186-204

146   Greenwood DC, Muir KR, Packham CJ, Madely RJ. Coronary heart disease: a review of the role of psycho-social stress and social support. *Journal of Public Health Medicine* 1996;18:221-231

147   Hillman M, Adams J, Whitelegg J. *One false move: a study of children's independent mobility*. London: Policy Studies Institute, 1991

148   British Medical Association. *Cycling: towards health and safety*. Oxford: Oxford University Press, 1991

149   See reference 114

150   See reference 114

151   National Centre for Risk Analysis and Options Appraisal. *Road transport and the environment. Risk Profile No 1*. London: Environment Agency, 1997

152   British Medical Association. *Water: a vital resource*. London: BMA, 1994

153   See reference 152

154   Office of Water Services. *Annual Report 1992*. London: HMSO, 1993

155   Ward N, Clark J, Lowe P, Seymour S. *Water pollution from agricultural pesticides*. Newcastle upon Tyne: Centre for Rural Economy, 1993

156   Cuninghame C, Griffin J, Laws S. *Water tight: the impact of water metering on low-income families*. London: Save the Children, 1996

157   See reference 54

158   See reference 54

159   See reference 22

160   Raphael A. *Ultimate risk*. London: Corgi Books, 1995

161   Corn JK. *Response to occupational heath hazards, a historical perspective*. New York: Van Nostrand Reinhold, 1992

162   See reference 160

163   Dalton AJP. *Health at work - should the HSE do more? Occupational Health Review* 1997;70:29-32

164   Office of Population Censuses and Surveys, and Health and Safety Executive. *Occupational health. Decennial supplement. The registrar general's decennial supplement for England and Wales. Series DS No 10*. London: HMSO, 1995

165   See reference 164

166   See reference 66

167   Morton S, Hannah J. Within minutes of the M62 - major retail development proposals for Greater Manchester. *Radical Community Medicine* 1989;38:28-34

168   Evans C A. Public health impact of the 1992 Los Angeles civil unrest. *Public Health Reports* 1983;108:265-272

169   Spongiform Encephalopathy Advisory Committee. *Statement* 24.3.96

170   Department of Health. *Monthly Creutzfeldt-Jakob Figures*. Press release 98/077. London: DoH, 1998

Chapter 5

1   Ashton J, Seymour H. *The new public health*. Milton Keynes: Open University Press, 1988

2   Draper P, Best G, Dennis J. *Health, money and the National Health Service*. London: Unit for the Study of Health Policy, Guy's Hospital Medical School, 1976

3   McKeown T. *The role of medicine - dream, mirage or nemesis?* London: Nuffield Provincial Hospitals Trust, 1976

4   British Medical Association. *Inequalities in health*. London: BMA, 1995

5   Townsend P, Davidson N, Whitehead M. *Inequalities in health*. London: Penguin, 1992

6   Benzeval M, Judge K, Whitehead M, eds. *Tackling inequalities in health: an agenda for action*. London: King's Fund, 1995

7   Scott-Samuel A. Health Impact Assessment. *BMJ* 1996;313:183-184

8   British Medical Association. *The BMA guide to living with risk*. London: Penguin Books, 1990

9   Department of Health. *Health of the Nation: Variations in Health*. London: HMSO, 1995

10   See reference 5

11   Brownlea A. From public health to political epidemiology. *Social Science and Medicine*. 1981;15D:57-67

12   Costongs C, Springett J. *A conceptual evaluation framework for health-related policies in the urban context*. Liverpool: Institute for Health, Liverpool John Moores University, 1995

13   Burdge RJ, Vanclay F. Social impact assessment. In: Vanclay F, Bronstein DA, eds. *Environmental and social impact assessment*. Chichester: John Wiley and Sons, 1995: 31-65

14   Interorganizational Committee on Guidelines and Principles for Social Impact Assessment. Guidelines and principles for social impact assessment. *Impact Assessment* 1994;12:107- 152

15   See reference 13

16   See reference 5

17   Wilkinson R G. Divided we fall. *BMJ* 1994;308:1113-4

18   Davey Smith G. Income inequality and mortality: why are they related? *BMJ* 1996;312:987-8

19   Scott-Samuel A. Unemployment and health. *The Lancet* 1984;2:1464-5

20   Bethune A. Economic activity and mortality of the 1981 Census cohort in the OPCS Longitudinal Study. *Population Trends* 1996;83:37-42

21   McGuire A, Henderson J, Mooney G. *The economics of health care. An introductory text*. London: Routledge and Kegan Paul, 1988

22   Begg D, Fischer S, Dombusch R. *Economics*. London: McGraw-Hill, 1984

23   Mishan EJ. *Cost benefit analysis*. London: George Allen and Unwin Ltd, 1971

24   Hutton J. Cost-benefit analysis in health care expenditure decision making. *Health Economics* 1992;1:213-216

25   Stirling A. Regulating the electricity supply industry by valuing environmental effects: how much is the emperor wearing? *Futures* 1992;24:10

26   Foster J, ed. *Valuing nature; economics, ethics and environment*. London: Routledge, 1997

27   Drummond M, Stoddart G, Torrance G. *Methods for the economic evaluation of health care programmes.* Oxford: Oxford Medical Publications, 1987

28   Johannesson M, Jonsson B. Economic evaluation in health care: Is there a role for cost-benefit analysis? *Health Policy* 1971;17:1-23

29   Sagoff M. *The economy of the earth: philosophy, law and the environment.* Cambridge: Cambridge University Press, 1988

30   See reference 25

31   O'Neill J. *Ecology, policy and politics.* London: Routledge, 1993

32   Office of Technology Assessment of the US Congress. *Studies of the environmental costs of electricity.* Washington DC: US Government Printing Office, 1994

33   See reference 26

34   Williams A, Kind P. The present state of play about QALYs. In: Hopkins A, ed. *Measures of the quality of life and the uses to which such measures may be put.* London: Royal College of Physicians, 1992

35   Mehrez and Gafni. Quality adjusted life years, utility theory and healthy year equivalents. *Medical Decision Making* 1989;9:142-149

36   Murray CJ, Lopez AD, Jameson DT. The global burden of disease in 1990: summary results, sensitivity analysis and future decisions. *Bulletin of the World Health Organisation* 1994;72:495-509

37   Torrance GW. Measurement of health state utilities for economic appraisal. *Journal of Health Economics* 1986;6:1-30

38   Mason J, Drummond M, Torrance G. Some guidelines on the use of cost-effectiveness league tables. *BMJ* 1993;306:570-572

39   Williams A. Economics of coronary artery bypass grafting. *British Medical Journal* 1985;29:326-329

40   Adapted from Williams A. Economics of coronary artery bypass grafting. *British Medical Journal* 1985;291:326-329

41   Sackett DL, Rosenberg WMC. On the need for evidence based medicine. *Health Economics* 1995;4:249-254

42   Mason J, Drummond M. The DH register of cost-effectiveness studies: quality and content. *Health Trends* 1995;27:50-6

43   Edwards RT, Boland A. *From "Health Services" Economics to "Health" Economics: Extending the scope of health economics to appraise the impact of non health sector policy on health.* London: Brunel Health Economics Study Group of Britain, 1996

44   Department of Health. *The health of the nation. A strategy for health in England.* London: HMSO, 1992

45   Department of Health. *Health of the nation: Fit for the future.* London: HMSO, 1995a

46   See reference 9

47   Department of Health. *Our Healthier Nation: Green Paper.* London: HMSO, 1998

48   See reference 47

49   Department of Health. *Policy appraisal and health, a guide for policy makers*. London: HMSO, 1995

50   Broome J. QALYs. *Journal of Public Economics* 1994;50:110-167

51   Carr-Hill RA, Morris J. Current practice in obtaining the Q in Qalys: A cautionary note. *BMJ* 1991;303:669-701

52   See reference 49

53   Birley MH. *The health impact assessment of development projects*. London: HMSO; 1995

54   Evans RG, Morris LB, Marmor TR, eds. *Why are some people healthy and others not? The Determinants of Health of Populations*. New York: de Gruyter, 1994

55   Ambrose P. *Bad housing - counting the cost*. Centre for Urban and Regional Research. Working paper No 90, 1996

56   Green J. *Housing, energy, health and poverty*. Paper presented at Healthy and Ecological Cities Congress. Madrid, 1995

57   See reference 43

58   See reference 54

Chapter 6

1   British Medical Association. *Pesticides, chemicals and health*. Edward Arnold: London, 1992

2   Ministry of Agriculture, Fisheries and Food. *The pesticides forum. Action plan for the responsible use of pesticides*. PF/5/Rev3. London: MAFF, 1997

3   Health and Safety Executive. Epidemiology and Medical Statistics Unit. *Feasibility study into the use of the National Proficiency Tests Council (NPTC) database of licensed agricultural pesticide users for epidemiological research*. London: HSE 1998

4   European Council of Chemical Manufacturers' Federations. *The chemical industry of western Europe: prepared for the 21st Century*. Brussels: CEFIC, 1986

5   British Medical Association. *Hazardous waste and human health*. Oxford: Oxford University Press, 1991

6   Office of Technology Assessment of the US Congress. *Serious reduction of hazardous waste for pollution prevention and industrial efficiency*. Washington DC: US Government Printing Office, 1986

7   Environmental Protection Agency of the United States. *Waste minimisation: environmental quality with economic benefits*. Washington DC: Environmental Protection Agency, 1987

8   See reference 5

9   Fingerhut MA, Halperin WE, Marlow DA, et al. Cancer mortality in workers exposed to 2,3,7,5-tetrachlorodibenzo-p-dioxin. *New England Journal of Medicine* 1991;324:212-8

10   See reference 5

11   See reference 5

12   British Medical Association. *Environmental and occupational risks of health care*. London: BMA, 1994

13   NHS Management Executive. *Occupational Health Services HSG (94)51*. London: Department of Health, 1994

14   NHS Management Executive. *Clinical Waste Management HSG (94)50*. London: Department of Health, 1994

15   Department of the Environment and the Department of Health. *The United Kingdom National Environmental Health Action Plan*. Cm 3323. London: HMSO, 1996

16   See reference 15

17   World Health Organisation. *Health and welfare Canada: Canadian Public Health Association (1986) Ottawa Charter for Health Promotion*. Copenhagen: WHO, 1986

18   Department of Health. *On the state of the public health, the Annual Report of the Chief Medical Officer of the Department of Health for the year 1994*. London: HMSO, 1995

19   Department of Health. *On the state of the public health, the Annual Report of the Chief Medical Officer of the Department of Health for the year 1995*. London: HMSO, 1996

20   Department of Health. *On the state of the public health, the Annual Report of the Chief Medical Officer of the Department of Health for the year 1996*. London: HMSO, 1997

21   Treweek JR, Thompson S. A review of the ecological mitigation measures in UK environmental statements with respect to sustainable development. *International Journal of Sustainable Development and World Ecology* 1997;4:40-50

22   Thompson S, Treweek JR, Thurling DJ. The potential application of SEA to the farming of Atlantic Salmon (Salmo salar L.) in mainland Scotland. *Journal of Environmental Management* 1995;45:219 229

23   Proposal for a Council Directive on the assessment of the effects of certain plans and programmes on the environment. COM/96/0511 Final - Syn 96/0304. *Official Journal of the European Communities*. No C129,25/4/97

24   Therivel R, Wilson E, Thompson S, Heaney D, Pritchard D. *Strategic environmental assessment*. London: Earthscan Publications Ltd, 1992

25   See reference 21

26   McCallum DP, Covello VT. What the public thinks about environmental data. *Environmental Protection Agency Journal* 1989:15;22-23

27   See reference 1

28   See reference 23

29   Department of Health. *Our Healthier Nation*: Green Paper. London: HMSO, 1998

30   Council Directive 97/11/EC of 3 March 1997 amending Directive 85/337/EEC on the assessment of the effects of certain public and private projects on the environment. *Official Journal of the European Communities*. No L073,14/3/97

31   Department of the Environment. *Environmental assessment: A guide to the procedures*. London: HMSO, 1997

32   Health and Safety (Emissions to the Atmosphere) Regulations 1983 (SI No.943)

33   Department of the Environment, Transport and the Regions. *Mitigation measures in environmental statements*. London: DETR, 1997

34   General Medical Council. *Recommendations on undergraduate medical education*. London: General Medical Council, 1993

Appendices

1   McMichael AJ. *Planetary overload. Global environmental change and the health of the human species*. Cambridge: Cambridge University Press, 1993

2   See reference 1

3   McKeown T. *The role of medicine - dream, mirage or nemesis?* London: Nuffield Provincial Hospitals Trust, 1976

4   World Health Organisation. *Concern for Europe's tomorrow: Health and the environment in the WHO European region. WHO European Centre for Environment and Health*. Stuttgart: Wissenschaftliche Verlagsgesellschaft, 1995

5   Department of Health. *The New NHS*: White Paper. Cm 3807. London: HMSO, 1997

6   Department of Health. *Our Healthier Nation*: Green Paper. London: HMSO, 1998

7   British Medical Association. Occupational Health Committee. *The occupational physician*. London: BMA, 1994

8   Department of the Environment. *The United Kingdom National Air Quality Strategy*. Cm 3587. London: HMSO, 1997

9   Department of the Environment. *Expert panel on Air Quality Standards - Benzene*. London: HMSO, 1994

10   Department of the Environment. *Expert Panel on Air Quality Standards - Nitrogen Dioxide*. HMSO: London, 1996

11   Kooijman JM. Environmental assessment of food packaging: impact and improvement. *Packaging Techology and Science* 1994;7:111-121

12   Bickerstaffe J, Turner B. *INCPEN Guide to the Boustead study on resource use and liquid food packaging 1986-1990*. London: INCPEN, 1993

13   See reference 12

14   Bullard B, Bender F. The packaging engineer's decision making process to assess packaging compatibility with the environment. Report produced for the PM Company Healthcare Group, Philadelphia, Pennsylvania, date unspecified

15   Sadler B. *International study of effectiveness of environmental assessment*. Canadian Environmental Assessment Agency and the International Association for Impact Assessment, 1996

16   Wood C. *Environmental impact assessment: A comparative review*. Harlow, Essex: Longman, 1995

17   Vanclay F, Bronstein D, eds. *Environmental and social impact assessment*. Chichester: Wiley, 1995

18   See reference 15

19 O'Riordan T, Sewell W, eds. *Project appraisal and policy review*. Chichester: Wiley, 1981

20 Caldwell L. Environmental impact analysis (EIA): origins, evolution and future directions. *Impact Assessment Bulletin* 1988;6:75-83

21 Keating M. *The Earth Summit agenda for change, a plain language version of Agenda 21 and the other Rio Agreements*. Geneva: Centre for Our Common Future, 1993

22 United Nations. *The global partnership for environment and development, a guide to Agenda 21 post Rio edition*. New York: United Nations, 1993

23 World Health Organisation. *Address by Dr H Mahler, Director-General of the World Health Organization in presenting his report for 1984 and 1985 to the Thirty-Ninth World Health Assembly, Geneva*. Geneva: WHO, 1986

24 World Health Organisation. *Health and safety component of environmental impact assessment. Environmental Health Series No. 15*. Copenhagen: WHO Regional Office for Europe, 1987

25 See reference 4

26 Birley MH. *Guidelines for forecasting the vector-borne disease implications of water resources development*. WHO/CWS/91.1. PEEM Guidelines Series 2. Geneva: World Health Organisation, 1991

27 Birley MH, Bos R, Engel CE, Furu P. Assessing health opportunities: a course on multisectoral planning. *World Health Forum* 1995;16:420 22

28 Birley MH, Bos R, Engel CE, Furu P. A multi-sectoral task-based course: Health opportunities in water resources development. *Education for Health: Change in Training and Practice* 1996;9:71-83

29 Cooper Weil DEC, Alicbusan AP, Wilson JF, Reich MR, Bradley DJ. *The impact of development policies on health: a review of the literature*. Geneva: WHO, 1990

30 World Health Organisation. *Commission on health and environment. Our planet, our health*. Geneva: WHO, 1992

31 Overseas Development Administration. *Manual of environmental appraisal. Revised edition*. London: Overseas Development Administration, 1992

32 Birley MH. *The health impact assessment of development projects*. London: HMSO, 1995

33 Birley MH, Peralta GL. *Guidelines for the health impact assessment of development projects*. Asian Development Bank Environmental Paper No 11, 1992

34 World Bank. *Environmental assessment sourcebook update, No 18 - Health aspects of environmental impact assessment*. Washington: World Bank, 1997

35 Listorti JA. *Bridging environmental health gaps - lessons from Sub-Sahara Africa infrastructure projects. Main Report, AFTES Working Paper No 20, Urban Environmental Management*. Washington: The World Bank, 1996

36 Bradley D, Stephens C, Harpham T, Cairncross S. *A review of environmental health impacts in developing country cities. Urban Management Program Discussion Paper 6*. Washington: The World Bank, 1992

37 Slooff R. *Commonwealth Secretariat Expert Group meeting on health impact assessment as part of environmental assessment*. Aberdeen, Scotland, 1995

38 See reference 34

39   See reference 17

40   Birley MH, Peralta GL. Health impact assessment of development projects. In: Vanclay F, Bronstein DA, eds. *Social and environmental impact assessment*. New York: Wiley and Sons, 1996

41   Konradsen F, Chimbari M, Furu P, Birley MH. The use of health impact assessments in water resource development: a case study from Zimbabwe. *Impact Assessment Bulletin*. In press

42   See reference 34

43   Ewan C, Young A, Bryant E, Calvert D. *National framework for health impact assessment in environmental impact assessment*. Australia: University of Wollongong, 1992

44   Public Health Commission. *A guide to health impact assessment. Guidelines for public health services and resource management agencies and consent applicants*. Wellington: New Zealand, 1995

45   Public Health Commission. *Risk assessment: A user friendly guide. Guidelines for public health services and resource management agencies and consent applicants*. Wellington: New Zealand, 1995

46   Kwiatkowski R. *The role of health professionals in environmental assessment, consolidated workshop proceedings*. Environmental Health Centre. Ottawa: Health Canada, 1996

47   Anon. *National health guide for environmental assessment: a discussion paper*. Prepared for the Federal-Provincial-Territorial Committee on Environmental and Occupational Health. The Environmental Health Centre. Ottawa: Health Canada, 1995

48   *EIA Newsletter 15*. Wood C, Barker AJ, Jones CE, eds. EIA Centre, Department of Planning and Landscape. University of Manchester, 1997

49   Aschemann und Jorde: *Umweltprüfung für Politiken Pläne und Programme - Untersuchung de Umsetzungsmöglichkeiten in Österreich*. Wien, 1996

50   Ordinance No. 97-1252. *Environmental Permits*. June 5, 1997

51   Ordinance No. 97-1253. *Organisation of Planning and Urban Development in the Brussels Capital Region*. June 5, 1997

52   Proposal for a Council Directive on the assessment of the effects of certain plans and programmes on the environment. COM/96/0511 Final - Syn 96/0304. *Official Journal of the European Communities*. No C129,25/4/97

53   Department of the Environment. *Sustainable development - a strategy for Ireland*. Dublin, Ireland: Department of the Environment, 1997

54   Arquiaga MC, Canter LW, Nelson DI . Integration of health impact considerations in environmental impact studies. *Impact Assessment*, 1994;12:175-197

55   Brantly E, Hetes R, Levy B, Powell C, Whiteford L. *Environmental health assessment: an integrated methodology for rating environmental health problems*. WASH Report 436, Office of Health and Nutrition, US Agency for International Development, 1993

56   Arcia G, Brantly E, Hetes R, Levy B, Powell C, Suarez J, Whiteford L. *Environmental health assessment: a case study conducted in the city of Quito and the county of Pedro Moncayo, Pichincha Province, Ecuador*. WASH report 401, Office of Health and Nutrition, US Agency for International Development, 1993

Index